# Healing with Herbal Juices

# Healing with Herbal Juices

*A Practical Guide to
Herbal Juice Therapy:
Nature's Preventative Medicine*

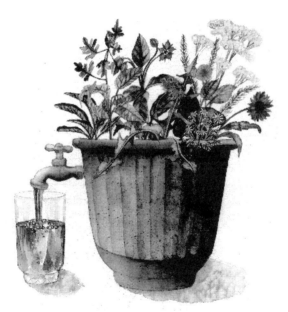

## Siegfried Gursche

Foreword by Zoltan P. Rona, MD, M.SC
Introduction by Keith Stelling, MH

books
Vancouver BC

*alive* books
PO Box 80055 Burnaby BC Canada V5H 3X1

Copyright © 1993 by Siegfried Gursche

Cover Design: Bill Stockmann
Cover Art: Irene Hannestad
Back Cover Photo: Ron Crompton
Typesetting: Sheila Adams

First Printing – June 1993


Canadian Cataloguing in Publication Data
  Gursche, Siegfried, 1933–
    Healing with herbal juices


    Includes bibliographical references and index.
    ISBN 0-920470-34-3

1. Vegetable juices–Therapeutic use. 2. Fruit juices–Therapeutic use.
3. Herbs–Therapeutic use. I. Title.
RM255.G87 1993      615.8'54 C93-091515-1

*Healing with Herbal Juices*
*is dedicated to my mother*
*who taught me all about life;*
*instilled in me a love for nature*
*and respect for all living things;*
*the value of live food*
*and how to live abundantly with little;*
*the happy side of life on earth*
*and the longing for life eternal.*

*An important scientific innovation rarely makes its way by gradually winning over and converting its opponents. What does happen is that its opponents die out and the growing generation is familiarized with the idea from the beginning.*

*Max Planck*

# Contents

Foreword     xi

Acknowledgements     xiii

Introduction     xv

I   Better Nutrition Through Freshly Pressed Juices     1

II   Medicinal Herbs Throughout History     11
    The popularity of medicinal herbs     13
    The secret of plant life     15
    Plant alchemy     17
    The meaning of natural therapy     20
    The Schoenenberger cellular plant juices     23
    Fresh-pressed cellular plant and herbal
       juices are different from other juices     26
    How to use fresh cellular plant juices     33

III   Nature's Gifts to Mankind     35
    **Acerola** – *the vitamin C powerhouse*     37
    **Artichoke** – *a natural liver tonic*     40
    **Asparagus** – *the weight loss gourmet*     42
    **Balm Mint** – *a most beloved and*
    **(Melissa)**    *versatile home remedy*     44
    **Bean (String)** – *a rare combination of*
       *effective ingredients*     46
    **Birch** – *the "blood" of the tree*     48
    **Black Radish** – *brings new life to both the liver*
       *and gallbladder*     50
    **Borage** – *increases your joy in living*     52
    **Camomile** – *the "wonder drug" of nature*     54
    **Carrot** – *the all-round vegetable*     56
    **Celery** – *an excellent dietary remedy*     58

**Coltsfoot** – *relieves asthma, bronchial catarrh,
        cough and loosens phlegm*                                60
**Dandelion** – *the incredible edible*                          62
**Echinacea** – *the immune system booster*                      65
**Fennel** – *a delightfully aromatic spice
        and medicinal herb*                                      67
**Fig Syrup** – *a truly "fruity" natural laxative*              68
**Garlic** – *the classic medicine*                              69
**Hawthorn** – *a heart tonic*                                   71
**Horseradish** – *a natural antibiotic*                         73
**Horsetail (Shave Grass)** – *a natural diuretic*               75
**Juniper** – *a natural antiseptic*                             77
**Mistletoe** – *a benefactor to your circulation*               79
**Oats** – *the best restorative for nervous exhaustion*         81
**Onion** – *a versatile home remedy through the millenia*       83
**Paprika** – *rich in vitamin C and a tonic
        for the heart and circulation*                           85
**Parsley** – *more than a culinary herb*                        86
**Plantain (Ribwort)** – *helps clear up mucus congestion*       87
**Potato** – *a benefactor to your stomach*                      89
**Pumpkin** – *the silent healer*                                91
**Ramson** – *a "wild" cousin of the garlic family*              93
**Red Beets** – *its multiple effects are still to be explored*  95
**Rosehips** – *five times more vitamin C than lemon*            97
**Rosemary** – *a natural stimulant for nerves
        and circulation*                                         99
**Sage** – *a saviour and healing mediator of nature*            100
**Sauerkraut** – *the best friend your digestive
        system could wish for*                                   102
**Silverweed** – *an anti-spasmodic juice*                       104
**Spinach** – *builds blood and restores cells*                  105
**St. John's Wort** – *strengthens your nerves*                  106
**Stinging Nettle** – *stimulates your metabolism*               108
**Thyme** – *a soothing anti-spasmodic*                          111

**Tomato** – *a harmonious set of vitamins*　　　113
**Valerian** – *soothing for the nerves*　　　115
**Watercress** – *the ideal spring tonic*　　　116
**Wormwood** – *a tried and true friend
　　　for over 4,000 years*　　　118
**Yarrow** – *improves the elacticity of
　　　blood vessels, strengthens muscles*　　　120

IV **Herbal Juice Therapies for Specific Ailments**　　　123
Arteriosclerosis Therapy　　　125
Arthritis and Rheumatism Therapy　　　128
Blood Purification Therapy　　　132
Circulation Therapy for Veins
　　and Low Blood Pressure　　　136
Circulation Therapy for High Blood Pressure
　　(Hypertension)　　　140
Female Complaints Therapy　　　142
Heart and Circulation Therapy　　　145
Kidney and Bladder Disorders Therapy　　　149
Liver and gallbladder Therapy　　　152
Nerve Restorative Therapy　　　155
Regenerative Therapy:
　　to raise your all-round energy level　　　159
Respiratory Tract Therapy – Colds,
　　Coughs, Sore Throat, Bronchial Catarrh　　　162
Slimming / Weight Reducing Therapy　　　166
Stomach and Intestinal Problems Therapy　　　174

V **Health Cocktails**　　　177
Natural "Pick-Me-Ups" For Feeling Better　　　179
　Anti-Flatulence Cocktail　　　182
　Beauty Cocktail　　　182
　Breathe-Easy Cocktail　　　183
　Cough Cocktail for Children　　　184
　Diuretic and Prostate Cocktail　　　184

Grippe Cocktail 184
Happy-Go-Lucky Cocktail 185
Heart's Delight Cocktail 185
Immune Booster Cocktail 186
Iron Supplementation Cocktail 186
Long Charlie Anti-Rheumatic Cocktail 187
Morning Health Cocktail 187
Relaxing Cocktail 188

**VI  A Final Word** 189
Perfect Health is Everyone's Right 191

**VII Appendices** 193
Appendix 1  Questions most often asked about
    herbal juices and therapies 195
Appendix 2  Important names in the
    history of medicine 199
Appendix 3  List of Botanicals 204
Appendix 4  Glossary of Therapeutic Terms 206
Appendix 5  Bibliography 209
Appendix 6  Useful Addresses 211

**Index** 213

**Tables**
Table 1  Presence of plant components
    by method of preparation 25
Table 2  Why cellular plant juices help 27

# Foreword

With so much of the health and medical industry focused on pills for ills, it's refreshing to read a book like *Healing with Herbal Juices*. This is not to say that drugs and nutritional supplements in the form of pills are a bad thing, but that a higher plane of healing can be found in herbal juice therapy. Herbal juice therapy is a safe alternative for many to use for prevention. It is also used as a form of complementary medicine for others already receiving conventional treatments.

We know that there are approximately 50 essential nutrients. Our bodies must get these from the diet in order to have optimal health. Since the standard North American diet fails to provide many of these nutrients for one reason or another, people have resorted to supplementation with pills containing vitamins, minerals, amino acids, herbs, enzymes and other food factors. But, can we really expect to get healthier with just supplements?

Nutritional medicine is in its infancy and many of the most respected experts in the field can only be said to be explorers of uncharted waters. For example, we know that plants contain many biologically active compounds that remain to be fully described. As Siegfried Gursche correctly points out, the conversion of plants or herbs into tablets, capsules and tinctures removes many of the vitamins, minerals and, in some cases, therapeutically active compounds. But what about the almost undiscovered therapy of herbal juices?

Siegfried Gursche has successfully distilled over 40 years of first-hand herbal experience with common ailments into this unique book. At one time, this sort of information was thought to be only anecdotal (unproven). Scientific research, however, is finally catching up to verify all the data you will find in the pages that follow. Medical doctors, and even groups such as the Canadian Cancer Society, are advocating things like vegetable juice as a source of the cancer preventative compound, beta carotene. Yet, beta carotene is only one of hundreds of beneficial compounds found in herbal juices.

You do not need an MD or PhD to understand or use the information in this book. What you will find here can be applied by anyone almost immediately. Herbal juice therapy is gaining prominence for many reasons. It's inexpensive. It's easily available. It's free of side effects if used correctly. This book shows you how. Lastly, it is based on the most up-to-date biochemical research. This is no longer esoteric knowledge used by the fringes of society, but a rapidly accepted mainstream way of becoming healthy and living longer in the twenty-first century. Modern disease prevention and therapeutics can no longer afford to do without it.

*Zoltan P. Rona, MD, MSc*
*Past President,*
*Canadian Holistic Medical Association*
*May 26, 1993*

# Acknowledgements

It started forty years ago. On the first day of my apprenticeship at a German health store called Reform Haus, my master, Friedrich Schulze, let me pick up the mail from the post office. An oversized letter with a postage meter impression caught my eye:

> *Von Magstadt geht Gesundheit aus*
> *In jede Stadt, in jedes Haus.*
> Meaning:
> From Magstadt, health and well-being spreads
> To every city, every home.

Magstadt, a small town in the Swabian Black Forest, is the home of Walther Schoenenberger's plant juice factory, where pure, fresh-pressed cellular herbal juices were made. These juices were not new to me as my mother used them whenever she didn't feel well – they kept her and our entire family healthy. But it was the simple slogan which made a lasting impression on me. Schoenenberger Plant Juices became part of my professional life.

I remember the couple who visited my own retail store in Vancouver on Fraser Street in 1954. They had heard that I imported herbal juices. The husband introduced me to his wife. She didn't look healthy – rather pathetic and timid. "Look at her," he said. "The doctors want to put her away. Essendale Clinic – electric shocks." The wife started crying, and he begged me to help her. She hadn't slept for almost a week.

I recommended two bottles of valerian juice, to calm her nerves, four bottles of St. John's Wort juice and a package of herbal sleeping tea – a three-week treatment. I suggested they try Kneipp's hydrotherapy treatment and a vegetarian raw food diet.

Four or five weeks later, when I had already forgotten the incident, a happy couple walked into my store. "Do you remember her?" the man asked. She beamed a smile that lit up her whole face. Tears rolled down her cheeks as she hugged me. They had come all the way from Abbotsford to thank me. This experience made another great impression on me, and confirmed my belief in Schoenenberger Plant Juices.

Had it not been for my mother, my master during my apprenticeship and my first customers, this book would never have been written.

Years later I visited the factory in Magstadt, and I was impressed to say the least. Walther Schoenenberger and his life's work have been a constant inspiration to me, and many years of study and practical experience have resulted in this book. I want to thank all those who have helped me with it. Rosalie Kani did numerous technical translations for me and offered her secretarial skills in typing the manuscript. Rebecca Clarkes, our first editor at *alive* magazine, did an extraordinary job in editing the first draft, while Marian MacLean helped in the final editing.

Several people have worked on this book through its stages, all helping to turn it into the finished product. Scott McDonald spent many hours at the computer inputting, and Annette Berndt provided proofreading and corrections. Gisela Temmel, managing editor, kept an eye on production schedules.

# Introduction

Herbal medicine is the oldest and most natural form of medicine and has been used safely and efficaciously for thousands of years. It is likely that the very first use of herbal medicine by mankind was in the form of fresh plant juices. But how could primitive man have found sophisticated juice extractors and how could he have prepared fresh plant juices without our modern mechanical and electrical methods? The answer is simple: he used his teeth.

Anyone who has spent time working in a herb garden will know how often one tends to break off a piece of leaf or stalk and quite unconsciously chew it for a quarter of an hour or more, until the fresh juice has ceased to please the tongue and the tasteless, tiresome fibres are spat out. For the North American Native people, as for all indigenous people around the planet, this natural juice extractor was the most common form of medicating and, except during the winter months when fresh plant material was not available and had to be used in dried form, it was the most widely used. Historical accounts indicate that the Indians living in present day Canada traded for Echinacea root with those living further south where the plant was a common weed. It is not hard to imagine them slowly chewing a piece of the root over the hundreds of miles of the homeward journey.

The early pioneers in Upper Canada were aware of the importance of using fresh plant extracts. An 1885 publication, *Medicinal Recipes of the late Doctor Taylor of Innerkip*, (Dr, Taylor was active in Southern Ontario from about 1820) stipulates that the root of the dandelion "loses much of its virtue by drying. It is mostly used in the form of extract which, of course, should be made from the fresh root. It acts more especially on the liver as a gentle stimulant and is valuable in torpor, inactivity and congestion of that organ, especially in chronic liver complaints. In such cases the extract is to be preferred and can be made from the fresh roots . . . ."

Although tinctures were developed in France in the late nineteenth century and have been used widely by professional herbal practitioners over the past 100 years, modern European phytotherapy is aware of the preference for the fresh extract of certain plants because of their greater biological activity. The famous French phytotherapist, Dr. Jean Valnet, as well as his predecessor, Henri Leclerc, specified on many occasions the need to use fresh plant material if optimum physiological effects were to be obtained. It appears that, with certain plants, some of the complex groups of constituents – sometimes as many as 170 different chemicals in a single plant – are either destroyed or inactivated during the drying process, rendering the plant material virtually ineffective. Although there are still a few "old-fashioned" herbalists who take great care to collect their own herbs from wildcrafted or organically grown specimens to make their own fresh plant extracts, harvesting them at precisely the time when essential oils are highest, for the most part, such quality medicine is no longer available commercially.

However, the Schoenenberger plant juices are an exception. For modern city dwellers who do not often have the opportunity of a long and leisurely chew of organic echinacea root as they travel on horseback through the sheltering glades of birch and pine forest, they are a Godsend. My first encounter with Schoenenberger plant extracts took place while I was still a student at the National Institute of Medical Herbalists' training clinic in London, England. It was undoubtedly through the enlightened thinking of the principal of the School of Phytotherapy, Hein Zeylstra, that they were part of the stock of our clinic dispensary. I still remember the first "miracle" I witnessed as a result of their use.

A fifty-six-year-old woman was brought into the clinic in a wheelchair. She had been suffering for five years from rheumatoid arthritis. Her swelling, immobility and depression were obvious. So too, was the frustration of some of the students of an earlier class who had had no success in treating her. "If only this patient could get out of the crowded city and experience the real healing power of nature," some of us thought.

The alternative was, of course, to bring nature into the city so someone decided to try the Schoenenberger juices, the closest to the live, growing herb that we could obtain. She was given birch *(Betula alba)* because of its diuretic properties and its reputation for removing uric acid from the tissues. Stinging nettle *(Urtica dioica)* was chosen because of the great wealth of trace minerals and vitamins it contains – vitamins A, $B_2$, C, K, iron, potassium and silica among others – as well as its eminent cleansing properties in arthritic conditions. We had been collecting nettles ourselves in the quiet countryside lanes around the herb farm where we were living, and had experienced noticeable benefit. And we were becoming aware that healing depended not only upon a list of chemical constituents in a plant – for example, the acetylcholine, the histamine or the beta carotene in nettles – but the whole combination of chemicals, and the environmental and spiritual dimension of the patient. If only this woman could also experience the sound of cuckoos, the warmth and quietness of the setting sun in the pasture with our two Jacob sheep, the smell of the pines and the hemlocks, and the other-worldly rhythm of the babbling stream that flowed past the seventeenth century mill house, there could be no question of her recovery. St. John's Wort was intended to take care of her depression by offering gentle nervine support and reducing some of the stress which was undoubtedly a result of constant pain. In addition, several other plants were used in tincture form, mainly to encourage circulation and to counteract inflammation.

The "miracle" was, of course, not instant, as real-life natural healing miracles seldom are; but the patient persisted with her treatment and her improved diet for several months, gradually achieving great relief from her pain. Eventually, she achieved enough mobility to journey out to the countryside to collect her own nettles. I remember seeing her a year later when, much to my astonishment, she was virtually recovered. She told us that she attributed the turning point in her progress to the introduction of the Schoenenberger plant juices into her treatment.

Central to all detoxification, and solidly underlying most herbal treatment, is the strategy of cleansing the liver as the central organ of elimination of the body, and at the same time restoring its ability to regulate dozens of distinct metabolic functions. Crucial to such therapy is one of the most dynamic natural remedies that has ever been discovered: the fresh leaves of the artichoke *(Cynara scolymus)*. In fact, it is almost a designer drug for the twentieth century. According to the Belgian Pharmaceutical Association's 1986 publication, *Compendium de Phytothérapie*, one of its constituents, cynarine, possesses intense choleretic properties which have been demonstrated clinically to significantly lower the cholesterol levels in the blood. While pharmaceutical drugs used for this purpose tend to induce reddening of the face and gastric irritation, artichoke is without secondary effects. The plant, therefore, finds a place in the treatment of atheroma. At the same time, it has been found to possess anti-hepatotoxic properties comparable to those of the milk thistle *(Carduus marianus)*.

Significantly, artichoke seems to be one of those plants that works best if it is used fresh. Schoenenberger artichoke juice fulfills this requirement quite nicely. It is widely used professionally for dermatological problems, and I suspect that my own clinical success in treating skin problems as stubborn as psoriasis and eczema is attributable, at least in part, to the fact that I always advise the sufferer to begin taking artichoke juice as a regular course of treatment, along with other herbal tinctures of my own making put together specifically for them.

But because treating hepatotoxicity takes precedence in all successful herbal treatment, it is not surprising that in recent years the Schoenenberger artichoke juice has played such an important role in strategies to revive those suffering from even the most serious degenerative diseases. Along with the freshly extracted juices of carrots and beets, it has been praised by a wide range of patients suffering from the side effects of conventional chemical therapy. Because there is no alcohol content to the Schoenenberger artichoke juice, it is the treatment of choice for liver impairment, especially when this has been brought about through immoderate consumption of alcoholic beverages.

The red beet *(Beta rubra)* is another pillar of liver treatment. One of its constituents, betaine, has been shown to be a regenerator of the liver when lipid levels are high and when it is affected by arteriosclerosis and circulation problems. The Belgian *Compendium* also suggests that current research on its cholin content indicates that it may be useful in treating tumors. Beet juice is widely employed by herbalists as a support to the immune system, and Valnet, in his *Traitment des Maladies par des Légumes, les Fruits et des Céréales* (1982) advised that the fresh juice can be taken with profit (a glass a day for a month at at time) in cases of anaemia, demineralization, anxiety, tuberculosis and even, (according to Dr. Ferenczi) cancer.

Borage *(Borago officinalis)* is another plant that is thought to lose its activity with drying. Its reputation as a "thymoleptic" or a remedy capable of lifting the spirits or counteracting depression, goes back to Elizabethan time. Yet a particularly modern concept is its application in adrenal exhaustion. It is favored by medical herbalists as part of a treatment to revive adrenal cortex function if it has been interrupted by long-term use of steroids.

These few examples illustrate the very real relevance of medicinal plants both in prevention of disease (and as a cost saving device for government health programs) and in supporting the body when it has been exposed to the destructive effects of powerful chemical drugs. The few I have mentioned are just the beginning of a whole harvest of remedies you will discover as you read this book.

Whether you are an ordinary citizen who has decided to take responsibility for your own health, or a health professional committed to the healing of those who seek your help, I strongly urge you to take note of what Siegfried Gursche so generously shares in the pages that follow. Your attention may be the turning point in a chronic illness and the beginning of a life of well-being.

*Keith Stelling*, MA, MNIMH, Dip. Phytotherapy

Keith Stelling is a member of the National Institute of Medical Herbalists of Great Britain, editor and founder of *The Canadian Journal of Herbalism*, a member of the Board of Editors of *The British Journal of Phytotherapy*, and a recent appointee to the Canadian government's Expert Advisory Committee on Herbs and Botanical Preparations. He is a lecturer in Botanical Medicine at the Canadian College of Naturopathic Medicine in Toronto and has his own busy herbal medicine practice in Stoney Creek, Ontario.

# I

# Better Nutrition Through Pressed Plant Juices

*Use them for vim, vigor and vitality!*

*Let food be your medicine
and your medicine be your food.*

*Hippocrates (470 - 377 BC)*

*Never doubt that a small group of thoughtful, committed citizens can change the world. It's the only thing that ever has.*

*Margaret Mead*

People are beginning to learn that they have the same responsibility toward their bodies as they do to a complex piece of machinery. They must ensure that their bodies are correctly adjusted, lubricated and in every way safe-guarded. Not to know our bodily requirements and fulfill them is to gamble with health. The World Health Organization defines health as "a state of complete physical, mental and social well-being, not merely the absence of disease or infirmity." Certainly health is much more than not being "sick in bed." There are degrees of "wellness," just as there are degrees of illness. Physical, mental and social well-being are interrelated.

Many people speak of food as "fuel for the engine." As a source of energy, food does have the same function as gas in a car, but it actually has far greater significance, since it is the material from which our bodies are rebuilt or regenerated. Every part of the body, even the bone structure, is in a constant process of wearing out, disintegrating and rebuilding. Therefore, food must constantly furnish the elements for regeneration.

Often the question is asked, "Can I enjoy the food I like and still be healthy?" One certainly can, provided food is chosen which will supply the ingredients necessary for regeneration of the worn-out cells. Nutrition scientists seem to be unanimous in agreeing that more than one half of all calories should come from raw vegetables, fruit and milk products. Life should be enjoyed, not endured. The prime of life can be extended and vigor retained through correct nutrition.

There is scope within the meaning of the term "nutrition," but if we consider it as a whole, we find that nutrition is nothing other than the flow of material substance through the architectural structure known as the "living organism" – from the moment at which life begins until the moment that life ceases. Since the whole of this structure is continuously being replaced by this flow, we can see that we are what we eat. In short then, everything we put through our mouth into our stomach makes a direct contribution to our physical well-being – or to our physical degeneration.

Fruits and vegetables have been recognized throughout the history of man as a natural source of the food substances needed to help protect the strength, vigor and youthful appearance most mature humans desire. At the beginning of creation God said, "Behold I have given you every plant yielding seed; it shall be food for you" *(Genesis 1:29)*. Fruit and vegetables were to be all that was eaten in the garden of Eden. However, much of the nutritional substances in these foods appear to be concentrated in their natural juices. These juices are "locked up," you might say, in the cellulose fibres of the plant, and in order to extract the nutrients the body must break down the fibrous cells. This is a major chore for some digestive systems, particularly for the elderly, whose problems may be further complicated by faulty teeth or dentures which cause difficulty in properly chewing fibrous foods.

In the interest of better health through easier digestion and assimilation, nutrition authorities recommend separating the juices from the fibrous materials *before* consuming. In this way, much of the nutritional benefit of a large amount of a fruit or vegetable may be obtained simply by drinking a few glasses of juice. We can, of course, drink *far more* juice than we can comfortably eat whole vegetables. About two kilos (4.4 lbs) of whole vegetables or fruit will make one half to one litre (approximately one quart) of juice. Naturally, the juice is a more concentrated form of the same nutritious and beneficial ingredients found in the whole vegetable, since only the cellulose is discarded. The juices, with all their minerals and vitamins, flood the body with materials to build strong, healthy cells. Thus, the body is revitalized in an amazingly short time through juice therapy. A person who has no time to eat a proper dinner can get all the nourishment he or she needs from a salad in the form of juice. Invalids and convalescents who have lost their appetite can drink their nourishment without having to force food into an unwilling stomach.

Those who suffer from stomach or intestinal ulcers often cannot eat raw vegetables, but they can easily drink soothing and healing carrot juice. Raw carrot juice is also excellent for babies. It can be mixed with milk without curdling and, because carrot juice provides the vitamins and minerals that give rich blood and good skin color, it is also invaluable for growing children. Besides, they will drink the naturally sweet juice when it is sometimes impossible to coax them to eat their vegetables. For adolescents, carrot juice aids the normal development of glands and helps to overcome acne.

Above all, raw vegetable juice taken daily by young and old, healthy and ill alike, guarantees that the body is receiving its quota of building material for its trillions of cells.

Walther Schoenenberger, a Swiss pharmacist, realized the healing and medicinal potential of fresh-pressed cellular plant juices early in this century. He also knew about the benefits to be derived from dried herbs and plants, but after reading and studying old herbal books, he saw that many of their medicinal ingredients were lost in the dehydration process. Earlier, more knowledgeable people had pressed their plants to obtain the maximum healing benefits.

Walther Schoenenberger devised a method of making and bottling fresh plant juices that preserved their medicinal qualities and their etheric oils so that people could use them year-round. In 1965, the German government impressed by what this one man had accomplished, awarded him a gold medal for his contributions to public health. Today, the

Schoenenberger fresh-pressed cellular juices are shipped from the factory in Magstadt, Germany to over 50 countries around the world, and you'll probably find them in your local health food store. Most of the therapies given in this book are the result of his clinical research.

You can, of course, press your own juices. Be certain to get freshly gathered plants, since they quickly deteriorate in storage. The plants must be grown in organically pure soil, free from chemical fertilizers, pesticides and herbicides. They should also be harvested at the exact moment when they contain the most medicinal ingredients. Pressing and bottling must be done under extremely sanitary conditions in order to avoid any bacterial contamination. You can be certain that these things are done with the juices pressed and bottled by Walther Schoenenberger. In the Black Forest and the Swabian Uplands the soil is extremely suitable for the growth of medicinal plants. In these nearly perfect conditions, far from traffic and pollution, most of the plants for the Schoenenberger juices are grown. They come under the daily supervision of scientists, who decide the right moment for harvesting and pressing.

Most of the crops are cultivated by local farmers under contract to the Schoenenberger plant juice works, and it is stipulated that no insecticides, chemical fertilizers or similar poisons are to be used. Through all stages of growth and production, both in the field and factory, the plants are under constant observation of trained scientists. Even after bottling, the juices remain under their watchful eyes until released for sale. With such rigid controls, the customer is guaranteed a juice of superior quality.

The proper pressing of juices is important. At the Schoenenberger factory it is done by experts using special equipment to extract all the valuable elements that are often carefully protected by nature within the complex fibrous cell structure. Hydraulic presses, designed by Walther Schoenenberger and his staff, are so efficient that not more than two to three hours elapse between harvesting and bottling. The hydraulic presses recover medicinal ingredients from the plant that the centrifuge type of home juicer is unable to. If you would like to press your own herbal juices, be sure to use a wheatgrass juicer.

Stinging nettle juice demonstrates that fresh-pressed plant juices are superior to the dried herb. As soon as you touch this plant, your skin is burned or "stung" by its etheric oil. Once the plant is cut and dried, this healing ingredient evaporates and the plant no longer stings. During the drying process the molecular structure of plants is changed: fermentation takes place and many valuable elements become insoluble and are no longer recoverable, even when prepared in tea form.

Only the fresh plant juice captures the whole synergistic complex of healing ingredients locked in the living plant. Walther Schoenenberger attributes the impressive therapeutic effects of plant juices not to any single substance, but to the complex effects of the various elements contained only in the fresh plant. His lifework motto is: "Keep what is natural as natural as possible." He also tells us that health is not a pill to be taken that remains in the body forever after. It is, in fact, an accomplishment which everyone must achieve for him or herself. But in this task man does not stand alone: nature has put a helping partner and friend at his side – namely, the plant. But it must be the whole plant: the natural biological unit.

Our ancestors knew the inexhaustible healing capacity of fresh plants. Wise men have passed on to us important knowledge and experience. Seldom, however, has anything so impressed Walther Schoenenberger as the following sentence, which is filled with simplicity: "The strength of your body lies in the juices of the plants." It sounds so topical that it is hard to believe its age, yet this quotation is more than 5,600 years old. The Chinese Emperor Shin-Nong (about 3,700 BC), more physician than ruler, and author of the oldest nature cure book in the world, used it to crown his life's work. We would do well today to listen to this ancient Chinese sage and to think again about the friends of our health – the plants – because in the past 150 years we have quite forgotten them. The pill, darling of an all-powerful chemistry-oriented empire, is acclaimed everywhere. Even the naturopathic profession has switched over to it and uses only the dried herb. According to Schoenenberger, herein lies much that is bad. In distancing ourselves from all that is natural, more and more of us see the real cause of the alarming and numerous diseases of our civilization.

When should we drink fruit and vegetable juices – and in what quantities? Before we consider that question, remember that nutritional authorities advise that juices should be consumed in as fresh a state as possible. Not only does exposure to air and continuous storage encourage nutrient loss, but fresh juices are more palatable.

So help get the day off to a good start: drink a large glass of freshly-made apple or orange juice before breakfast. Then have a large glass of vegetable juice mixtures, either in the middle of the morning or before the evening meal, and again as a nightcap. There is nothing finer than a drink of fresh-pressed juice before retiring.

One of North America's most prominent pioneers of fresh juice was Gayelord Hauser. In a sanatorium in Carlsbad, Czechoslovakia, he discovered first-hand the immense healing and invigorating power of raw juices. "Since then," he states, "I have recommended a daily pint of fresh vegetable juice to every human being I have met. I am convinced, after all these years, that the addition of one pint of vegetable juice to the daily diet is one of the best safeguards against tiredness and premature aging."

In the same sanatorium, Gayelord Hauser heard for the first time about the green magic of chlorophyll in plants. Vegetable juices, he argues, are literally the "blood of the plant," poured out to serve of mankind in the healing of diseases and the restoration of health. For example, it was a time of great excitement in California in the early 1960s when Dr. Cheney announced that fresh cabbage juice cured ulcers in two weeks! His cure was based on giving his patients one litre (one quart) of fresh cabbage juice, or 75 percent cabbage and 25 percent celery juice. It was the first time fresh vegetable juices were officially recognized on this continent. But why only cabbage or celery juice? *All* fresh juices have marvellous healing powers, not only because of their vitamin and mineral content, but because of the *matière vivante*, as Dr. Bircher-Benner from Switzerland called it – and no chemist has yet been able to duplicate this energy.

When making juices at home, it is best to use an electric juicer of either the centrifugal type for hard fruits and vegetables or the expeller type, such as the Champion juicer, which makes it possible to extract the juice from soft fruit and berries. Both types are unsuitable for pressing juice from herbs. A meat grinder type berry press or a wheatgrass juicer allows you to press fresh herbal juice.

Schoenenberger juices have several advantages over home-pressed juices. The plants are guaranteed to be organically grown and harvested at their peak, ensuring the best medicinal value. They are pressed hydraulically within a few hours of harvesting and bottled under extremely sanitary conditions, preventing any bacterial contamination. Once sealed, their potency has no time limit. When opened though, these natural, fresh-pressed juices must be kept in the refrigerator and used within a short period (eight to ten days) in order not to lose the inherent medicinal ingredients.

The choice is entirely yours – either make your own juices daily from extremely fresh, organically grown produce, or buy them from the health store. Whatever you decide, make sure juices are part of your daily health routine.

The experiments and research of dieticians, nutritionists, naturopaths and scientists have brought about many new insights into proper nutrition. The therapies outlined in this book are the result not only of modern scientific medical-pharmaceutical achievements, but also of our ancient medical heritage and folk knowledge of plants and medicinal herbs.

In this technological century, man is gradually becoming aware of the mutual interrelations and interdependence of all creation. This new awareness also brings into sharp focus how much man has become alienated from nature in general, especially in his neglect of natural foods and the healing properties found in plants, herbs and fruits. Research into past traditions, cultures, folklore and ancient remedies from old herbal books has brought to light not only a wealth of "sensible" knowledge, but many confirmations by twentieth century chemists and scientists: the findings of our forefathers, though often based on "mere feelings" and observations, were basically correct, and in many instances even ahead of present knowledge.

In this book, an attempt has been made to investigate further the results of this research by tracing medicinal herblore throughout history, and by providing a cross-section of medicinal herbs and plants, and plant juice therapies. May it open the eyes of all who wish to better safeguard their health – the greatest treasure in this world.

# II

# Medicinal Herbs
# Throughout History

*All men ought
to be acquainted
with the medical art.*

*Hippocrates (470 - 377 BC)*

*Through the centuries,*
*healing has been practiced*
*by folk-healers who are guided*
*by traditional wisdom that sees illness*
*as a disorder of the whole person.*

*Prince Charles*

# The Popularity of Medicinal Herbs

We are witnessing a remarkable turning point in the history of the healing sciences. It seems that purely science-oriented medicine, based on the treatment of symptoms alone – a "materialistic" period of healing – is coming to an end. The tremendous wealth of experience gained by physicians through many centuries – even millennia – is now seen in a new light. The more progressive thinkers in the field of modern medicine are already building bridges between the present healing methods and those of previous epochs in order to ensure a more encompassing, firm foundation for the healing sciences of the future.

There is no need and no intention to belittle the great accomplishments and successes of science-oriented medicine which achieved its highest peak at the turn of the twentieth century. Many valuable new tools and methods enlarged the scope of every single physician. But at the same time, these incredible achievements and inventions of electronic equipment have led to an arrogance of attitude which considers the present medical plateau beyond criticism. Yet, more and more people are not satisfied with a treatment that emphasizes drugs that cause unpleasant side effects. The cry of "Back to nature and natural healing methods!" is steadily growing in intensity and volume.

The old herbalists produced cures equal to anything achieved by modern medicine and, because of their knowledge, their "simple" herbal remedies rarely caused harmful side effects or other disorders. Present-day pharmaceutical chemists, of course, continue to use plants for medicinal purposes. "The trouble is that they believe they are doing the right thing, and being scientific by isolating what they call the 'curative principle' of a herb, giving the extract an impressive title and marketing it as a new drug. Often these extracts are blended with minerals and other drugs," states Eric F. W. Powell, ND.[1] However, when a curative principle is taken out of its natural setting, in the plant, it actually *loses* some of its effectiveness and can even be detrimental to one's health. Such isolated extracts are not nearly as medicinally reliable as the entire plant.

Nature always provides her healing and nourishing elements as a complex whole. For instance, the B vitamins are completely interrelated, and in any food where one B vitamin is found, others are there as well. An isolated B vitamin is of little benefit to the body. It must work together synergistically with other B vitamins. In fact, too much of one B vitamin will use up the other Bs and create a deficiency, which is why a B complex intake should always be balanced and in its natural state, as it is in grains and brewer's yeast. Similarly, vitamin C, a constituent of citrus fruits, green pepper and rosehips among others, is always linked with the bioflavonoids.

Freshly pressed cellular juices are a concentrated form of elements preserved as a whole complex, just as nature intended. Because they are so complete, these plant juices are far superior to isolated medicinal ingredients or drug derivatives.

---

[1] Powell, Eric F. W., ND., *About Dandelions. The Golden Wonder Herb*, p 7.

## The Secret of Plant Life

For centuries man has attempted to lift the veil which hides the secret of plant life, but still has not quite removed it. While Aristotle's statement that "plants have souls but no sensation" was accepted as dogma throughout medieval times, right up into the eighteenth century, Carl von Linné, the grandfather of modern botany, claimed that plants differ from humans and animals only by their lack of movement. Then the nineteenth century botanist Charles Darwin proved that every tendril has its own power of independent movement. But as Darwin put it, "plants acquire and display this power only when it is of some advantage to them." Raoul Francé, a Viennese biologist, shocked the natural philosophers at the beginning of the twentieth century with his idea that plants move their bodies as freely, easily and gracefully as the most skilled human or animal. The only reason we don't appreciate the fact, he argued, is that plants do so at a much slower pace.

According to Francé, the roots of plants burrow inquiringly into the earth, buds and twigs swing in definite circles, leaves and blossoms bend and shiver with change, and tendrils stretch out inquiringly to feel their surroundings. We think of plants as both motionless and without feeling because we don't take time to watch them, but various kinds of electronic tests done in the past 25 years – not to mention the Kirlian photography of plant plasma – indicate that plants radiate energy.

Paracelsus, the "Swiss Hermes" of the fifteenth century, wrote extensively about herbs and "their secret virtues."

Through reading the works of European herbalists and the wise men of the Middle East – and primarily from his own observation and study of nature – Paracelsus became one of the most knowledgeable men of all time about the use of medicinal plants.

Therapy was always uppermost in the thinking of Paracelsus, and should be based, he argued, on the "law of affinities," once the causes of disease had been ascertained and eliminated. He also recognized the importance of nutrition, and to him, food was not merely a physical substance – it was a medium for the transmission of energy.[1]

---

[1] Hall, Manly P., *The mystical and medicinal properties of Paracelsus*, p 13.

# Plant Alchemy

Inorganic minerals were never intended to be used as medicine; the digestive and assimilative systems are designed to deal only with organic substances. All the mineral matter the body requires is supplied in an "organized" form in plant life. These nutritional substances can be absorbed and assimilated completely by the human body. Crude minerals may be partially absorbed, but this is not the same as assimilated. Only what is completely absorbed enters the tissue cells. Foreign substances may be either eliminated in due course, or remain in the intercellular spaces, eventually to become a type of growth to clog and obstruct organic function.

Mineral matter, as found in plant life, is essential to every function in the body. It is not enough to supply protein and starches and attend only to the fueling of the organism. Thinking and reasoning would not be possible without the minerals called *phosphates*, and communication between mind and body would cease. Without calcium and silica the bones and teeth would crumble into decay, and if sodium did not enter into our food, digestion and assimilation would come to a grinding halt. Indeed, it may be said that every mineral element found in the earth is also found in man, even in very minute traces, and each has a part to play. This is true of gold, silver, copper, zinc, tin, magnesium and all other more rare elements. Traces are also to be found in plants and vegetables, especially in wild growth where human chemicalization and errors have not interfered. Some of these elements are found in our systems in such minute quantities that they would not cover the tip of a single finger nail – yet they are essential.

In 1873 a Hanoverian baron, Albrecht von Herzeele, published a revolutionary book, *The Origin of Inorganical Substances*, which offers proof that, far from simply absorbing substances from the soil and the air, living plants are continuously creating matter. During his lifetime, von Herzeele made hundreds of analyses indicating that the original content of potash, phosphorus, magnesium, calcium and sulphur quite inexplicably increased in seeds that were sprouted in distilled water. Von Herzeele's analyses proved also that not only mineral ash, but every one of the plant's components, such as nitrogen, increased and burned off during incineration of the seeds. All this occurred in spite of the law of the conservation of matter: that exactly the same mineral content in plants grown in distilled water would be found in the original seeds. Thus the baron discovered the ability of plants to transmute, in alchemical fashion, phosphorus into sulphur, calcium into phosphorus, magnesium into calcium, carbonic acid into magnesium, nitrogen into potassium and silica into iron.

These extensive experiments were checked out quite recently by Pierre Baranger, professor and director of the Laboratory of Organic Chemistry at the famous École Polytechnique in Paris. He himself was astounded at the results when he announced his discoveries to the scientific world in January 1958 at Switzerland's *Institut Genevois*, concluding: "There is no way out. We have to submit to the evidence. Plants know the old secret of the alchemists. Every day under our very gaze they are transmuting elements."[1]

By now, at the end of the twentieth century, both Russian and American scientists agree. "The time has come to recognize that any chemical element can turn into another, under natural conditions," claims P. A. Korolkov of the former

---

[1] Tomkins, P. and Bird, C., *The secret life of plants*, p 290.

USSR.[2] "This offers a totally different approach to our understanding of nutritional supplementation, of the elements, and how they function in the physiological and biochemical pathways of our bodies," concurs Dr. Michael Walczak of California. "It attempts to prove that our concepts of simple supplementation for deficiencies is not only questionable, but in serious error."[3]

As we can see, today's scientists, chemists and nutritionists are subjecting old folklore and the wisdom of medieval herbalists to the scrutiny of microscopes and laboratory tests, only to arrive at the very same results! Further research has shown that the lack of trace elements in soils and in foods leads to an imbalance in enzyme function. Michael Walczak, MD says he is preventing and curing diseases by administering the right amount of enzymes, hormones, vitamins and minerals, which together he calls "the key to life." He concludes that the "gold," which the medieval chemists tried to derive from lead, may well turn out to be the secret for obtaining good health and long life.

---

[2] Korolkov, P. A., *Spontaneous metamorphism of minerals and rocks*, 1972.
[3] Walczak, V. Michael MD., *Study on Kervan's natural transmutations*.

# The Meaning of Natural Therapy

We are already aware that where health is concerned there exists an extreme dissatisfaction. At the moment, this dissatisfaction is directed against the use of dangerous drugs, chemicals in foods, "factory farming" of land and many other instances of "progressive civilization." However, it is also the general consensus that this fight against the tide of dangerous drug therapy and the chemicalization of food and soil does not, by itself, ensure an improved standard of health. In addition to the proper direction and co-ordination of such a movement there is the paramount need to find a positive alternative to the established, orthodox system of medicine. Natural therapies using natural herbal and plant remedies fill that need.

Natural therapy is a positive approach to disease. It postulates a way of life that considers the whole person, not just the symptoms. Natural therapy is preventative medicine in its most efficient and scientific form, based on the concept that "only nature heals" and that within the human organism lies the essential healing power to overcome disease. "Leave it to nature" is still a common expression. Hippocrates, the father of medicine, said, "Nature alone heals," and this contention has stood the test of time.

Man was created a healthy unit. As long as he observes the natural laws for which his body was designed, he remains a healthy unit – even unto death. Unfortunately, as civilization progressed, the observance of natural laws receded, and many of the consequences we have come to are accepted as inevitable.

The degeneration of food, land and animals has assumed such alarming proportions that now public pressure is demanding a return to more natural methods of living. Somewhere, somehow, an answer to this problem must be found – one that is compatible with a modern society. Natural therapy offers most of the answers.

As he regresses from natural laws, we inevitably find that man becomes a sickly being and his sickness grows with each violation of the laws he was constructed to observe. The resilience of man is both one of his virtues and one of his weaknesses. Without this inherent tendency to be healthy, man would probably have rendered himself extinct by now. It is this very tendency which the orthodox drug user suppresses and which the naturopath encourages. Naturopathy (natural therapy) recognizes that disease is the result of the violation of natural laws. Individually, we eat too much, drink too much and similarly indulge in the addictive, so-called pleasures of tobacco and alcohol. Our lives soon reveal patches of "sub-health" and illness because of this self-indulgence. At this stage we resort to drugs which, unfortunately, only suppress the symptoms of the disease, deluding us into assuming that health is once more with us. But this is not so – and no one is more aware of it than the naturopath. The medical profession should also be cognizant of the fact that real health is on the decline. The annual statistics that reveal the growing incidence of rheumatism, arthritis, nerve disorders, heart disease and cancer, point to the failure of orthodox medicine to recognize the direct link between nutrition and degenerative diseases.

Natural therapy, therefore, insists that disease is created by the departure from the natural laws that govern diet, exercise, sun, fresh air and environment. When these natural laws are obeyed, health follows. Obviously, the curing of disease calls for the application of methods that will assist the healing power of the body. Such methods are fasting, diet, water treatments, the use of sun and air, biological medication, exercise and manipulation, electrotherapy, herbal remedies and, above all, the use of pure, natural, fresh-pressed cellular plant and herbal juices.

It is in connection with the latter that Walther Schoenenberger was decades ahead in his research. He utilized the wisdom of times gone by and submitted those findings to the tests and processing methods of modern medical-pharmaceutical technology. It is in this area that he is an outstanding pioneer, a forerunner who has anticipated our present needs and predicaments. His pure, natural-pressed plant and herbal juices, so conveniently bottled to last an indefinite time while conserving full potency, are part of the positive alternative to the established negative system of healing.

These plant and herbal juices are proof of Walther Schoenenberger's deep intuitive insight into the interrelatedness of natural plant organisms and their destined value for mankind. It is from this point of view that one has to understand the success of the pure, natural-pressed plant and herbal juices; it is not to be approached as a "prescription." The use of plant juices presents a challenge to the true calling of a physician who does not follow routine alone, but combines observation and an inner receptiveness with his or her knowledge of natural laws. In short, it calls for an appreciation of the wholistic approach to both the art of healing and to the patient.

# The Schoenenberger Cellular Plant Juices

Walther Schoenenberger claimed plant juice therapy to be a new path in herbal treatment – a highly specialized system designed to wage war on the many ills and complaints of this nerve-jarring age. His laboratory experiments proved that dried herbs had an altogether different consistency and quality from fresh herbs and the juices of fresh herbs because the fermentation and oxidation processes bring about significant changes *(see Table I)*. Drying is actually a wilting of the plant, and wilting implies loss of water and disturbance of the life structure. Subsequent moistening cannot recapture the original condition, as evidenced by soaking dried apples or plums. By the same token, all fluid extracts, whether in a water or an alcohol base, forsake certain components inherent only in fresh plant cell juices. The *fresh plant* is a single harmonious whole, a biological unit, for which Walther Schoenenberger had the highest respect and admiration. He handled plants with great reverence. "To add nothing and to take nothing away," was his rule when dealing with herbs. It never entered his mind to create a new healing system. All he wanted was to maintain those already available, "just as nature created them."

A healing therapy which is truly allied to nature should be directed to the ailing body as a complete unit. It is not a single organ that is sick, but the whole person. Fresh, cellular plant juices do not fight symptoms or relieve a single complaint. Rather, they are able to steer the entire functioning of the human body onto natural and healthy paths.

Combinations of Schoenenberger juices are especially prepared for specific illnesses, whether of the liver, the kidneys, the stomach, the intestines, the heart or the circulation. The synergistic effect of the active substances of these juices is well known and scientifically proven. Walther Schoenenberger holds the view that *each plant is a complex structure of elements*. A particular element is not only dependent on all others, but can only release its full effective essence when *all* elements work together in the biological unit of the fresh plant. This he calls the "active substance cycle" of the plant, which works extraordinarily well on the complex body system of man. Under no circumstances should that cycle be broken.

According to the latest scientific tests, certain important effective ingredients cannot be dissolved and isolated from the plant without risking modification to the delicate plant structure. Furthermore, it has been shown that many elements in the fresh plant up to now considered unimportant, play a very important role in the maintenance of our bodily functions. There is, for example, the yellow pigment especially abundant in wild herbs. It has now been ascertained that this yellow pigment has two important tasks to fulfill simultaneously: to regulate the permeability of cell membranes and to assist in the process of mineral transmutation.

## Table I

*Presence of plant compounds by method of preparation*

| Component | Dried Herb | Tincture | Juice |
| --- | --- | --- | --- |
| **albumen** | present in small amounts | not present | present in natural form |
| **sugars** | present but changed | present but changed | present in natural form |
| **pigment** | present but changed | present but changed | present |
| **bitters** | present but changed | present | present in natural form |
| **starch** | scarcely detectable | – | present in natural form |
| **tannin** | present but changed | present but changed | present in natural form |
| **original biological water** | – | – | present |
| **minerals** | partly present | scarcely detectable | present in organic form |
| **etheric oils** | scarcely detectable | partly present | present |
| **vitamins** | present in small amounts | not found | present in natural form |
| **trace elements** | present | not found | present in organic form |

It is quite apparent that loss or change in the quality of the inherent ingredients in common preparations is considerable when compared to the fresh cellular plant juices.

## Fresh-Pressed Cellular Plant and Herbal Juices are Different from Other Juices

First of all, the body's acceptance and assimilation of the elements is facilitated with cellular plant juices because they correspond to the original, natural solution within the plant cells. (Remember, there is a basic affinity between man and the kingdom of plants, particularly in the correspondence of our blood to the chlorophyll in the plant juice.)

Secondly, the organically conditioned mildness of the juices, in contrast to the strong concentrates of chemical medications, is gentle to the stomach and intestines. The complete removal of all burdensome cellulose-fibre parts of the plant make the plant juices particularly acceptable to even the most debilitated and sensitive digestive tract.

Thirdly, the versatile organic components of the plant combine with mineral substances drawn from the soil to build a natural, whole entity. In this completeness, the plant's ingredients unfold with a more harmonious effectiveness than from any single isolated component.

Finally, as all fresh cellular plant juices contain a preponderance of minerals, they will invariably counteract any over-acidity in the blood. In other words, these juices will restore the correct mineral balance.

The following table lists briefly the juices which are particularly effective for specific complaints. However, such a brief synopsis is not meant to detract from, or add to, the juices' place in the framework of cellular plant juice therapy.

# Table II
## *Why cellular plant juices help*

| When to use | Which Juice(s) | Why |
| --- | --- | --- |
| **Asthma** (breathing problems) | coltsfoot juice plantain (ribwort) juice thyme juice horsetail juice St. John's Wort juice onion juice | coltsfoot loosens mucus, plantain is an anti-inflammatory, thyme is for croupy coughs, horsetail's silicic acid strengthens tissues, St. John's Wort is for breathing difficulties, onion juice is for colds and mucus in the upper respiratory tract |
| **Aging** | artichoke juice hawthorn juice | artichoke juice lowers cholesterol in the bloodstream and hawthorn juice strengthens the heart |
| **Anemia** (iron deficiency) | nettle juice spinach juice | contain iron, plus specific vitamins and elements for building blood cells |
| **Arteriosclerosis** | garlic juice or ramson juice plus hawthorn juice or mistletoe juice | garlic and ramson juices promote circulation and ease the discomforts of arteriosclerosis, hawthorn juice helps the heart and regulates blood pressure |
| **Arthritis** (inflammation of the joints) | celery juice horseradish distillate (over a period of time) | diuretic properties work through the kidneys |
| **Back Pain** (lower back) | yarrow juice horsetail juice celery juice | yarrow and horsetail juice strengthen tissue and muscle, celery juice is a diuretic |
| **Bad Breath** | wormwood juice | cleanses stomach and aids digestion |
| **Bladder Catarrh** | horsetail juice birch juice parsley juice | horsetail strengthens tissues and is an anti-inflammatory, birch cleanses kidneys (renal passages), parsley stimulates kidney functions |
| **Blood Congestion** (head rush) | hawthorn juice yarrow juice | hawthorn eases pressure, regulates and strengthens circulation, yarrow is an anti-spasmodic and tranquilizing agent |

| When to use | Which Juice(s) | Why |
|---|---|---|
| **Blood Building** | spinach juice | high content of vitamins for building blood cells |
| **Blood Pressure** (high) | garlic juice<br>hawthorn juice | garlic lowers blood pressure and serum cholesterol levels, hawthorn strengthens heart functions |
| **Blood Pressure** (low) | hawthorn juice | normalizes blood pressure by facilitating heart action and by directly influencing blood vessels |
| **Blood Purification** | nettle juice<br>dandelion juice<br>celery juice | nettle juice helps the metabolism, dandelion juice mobilizes toxins, celery juice is a diuretic |
| **Blood Vessels** (strengthening) | acerola juice | vitamin C and bioflavonoids strengthen the finer blood vessels |
| **Bronchial Asthma** | coltsfoot juice<br>horsetail juice<br>(over a period of time)<br>St. John's Wort juice | coltsfoot loosens phlegm, horsetail tones up the respiratory system, St. John's Wort soothes the nerves |
| **Bronchial Catarrh** | coltsfoot juice<br>plantain (ribwort) juice<br>horsetail juice | coltsfoot (an expectorant) loosens phlegm, plantain is an anti-inflammatory, horsetail contains silicic acid and helps the respiratory system, strengthens tissues |
| **Cholesterol** (elevated serum level) | artichoke juice<br>birch juice | artichoke lowers cholesterol levels, birch stimulates kidney functions, and helps eliminate uric acid |
| **Circulation**, poor | hawthorn juice<br>yarrow juice<br>bean juice | hawthorn strengthens heart muscle and circulation, yarrow is a relaxing anti-spasmodic, bean is a diuretic |
| **Constipation** (or tendency to irregularity) | fig syrup | fig sugar promotes movement of the large intestine |
| **Convalescence** | red beet juice<br>red beet powder | red beet juice, rich in iron, enriches blood and hemoglobin |

| When to use | Which Juice(s) | Why |
| --- | --- | --- |
| **Coughs** | coltsfoot juice<br>plantain (ribwort) juice<br>thyme juice<br>fennel juice | coltsfoot juice loosens phlegm, plantain (ribwort) juice soothes inflammation, thyme juice relaxes, cleanses and disinfects bronchial passages, fennel loosens phlegm |
| **Cramps and Spasms** | yarrow juice<br>silverweed juice | yarrow relaxes and dilates blood vessels, silverweed supports the action of yarrow juice synergistically and acts as a restorative |
| **Cystic Catarrh** | horsetail juice<br>birch juice | stimulate and strengthen the kidneys |
| **Diarrhea** | yarrow juice | spasm relieving element in yarrow juice |
| **Dieting** | artichoke juice<br>nettle juice<br>potato juice<br>tomato juice<br>asparagus juice | artichoke provides bitters and stimulates liver functions, nettle juice stimulates metabolism, potato and tomato juice provide valuable minerals, eliminate acids and metabolic waste, asparagus prevents water retention |
| **Digestive Disorders** | sauerkraut juice<br>wormwood juice<br>nettle juice<br>fig syrup | sauerkraut juice regulates intestinal flora, wormwood juice aids the stomach, nettle juice aids elimination, fig is a purgative |
| **Diuretic Problems** | celery juice<br>bean juice | potassium salts and etheric oils in both juices have a diuretic effect |
| **Exhaustion** | oat juice<br>rosemary juice | fortifying elements contain nitrogen, stimulate circulation |
| **Female Complaints** (menopause and menstruation problems) | borage juice<br>yarrow juice | borage juice is a tonic for the timing of hormonal activity, yarrow juice controls a thumping heart, quickened pulse, giddiness and head noises, has a regulatory effect on blood vessels, silverweed is an antispasmodic |

| When to use | Which Juice(s) | Why |
|---|---|---|
| **Fever** | red beet juice<br>acerola juice | red beet juice strengthens the immune system and supplies iron, acerola promotes resistance by supplying vitamin C and provitamin A |
| **Flatulence** | yarrow juice<br>fennel juice | spasm-relieving elements in yarrow and relaxing aromatics (etherical oils) in fennel |
| **Gall Bladder Complaints** | black radish juice<br>dandelion juice | the etheric oils and magnesium in black radish juice stimulate the liver and promote the flow of gall, in combination with dandelion juice it inhibits the formation of gallstones |
| **Gastric Catarrh** | wormwood juice<br>yarrow juice | wormwood juice is a stomach tonic, yarrow soothes and relieves spasms |
| **Glands**<br>(underactive, spleen, liver, gallbladder) | nettle juice<br>parsley juice<br>watercress juice | nettle stimulates metabolism, parsley stimulates and strengthens digestive system, watercress has a cleansing, restorative, stimulating effect |
| **Gum Infection** | sage juice (mouthwash)<br>camomile juice | sage juice disinfects and strengthens, camomile juice is anti-inflammatory |
| **Headaches** | wormwood juice<br>hawthorn juice<br>parsley juice | wormwood juice helps the stomach and is effective where the cause of headache or migraine lies in the stomach, hawthorn juice promotes circulation, parsley juice affects blood vessels |
| **Heart Trouble**<br>(nervous origin) | hawthorn juice<br>yarrow juice<br>valerian juice | hawthorn increases blood flow to the heart, helps its function, normalizes the fluctuation in blood pressure, yarrow cleanses the blood vessels |
| **Heartburn**<br>(caused by overacidity) | potato juice | potato juice lowers the activity of the stomach glands and secretion rate of stomach digestive juices |
| **Hoarseness** | plantain (ribwort) juice<br>sage juice | plantain (ribwort) juice relieves inflammation, sage juice disinfects and should also be used as a gargle |

| When to use | Which Juice(s) | Why |
|---|---|---|
| **Hyperactivity** | valerian juice | calms the nervous system |
| **Immune system** | echinacea juice | strengthens the immune system |
| **Infections** | echinacea juice | inhibits inflammation, disinfects, promotes wound healing |
| **Insomnia** | valerian juice | extremely calming and sleep inducing, even after prolonged use without side or after effects |
| **Intestinal Detoxification** | garlic juice<br>sauerkraut juice | garlic normalizes intestinal flora, kills bacteria, sauerkraut regulates intestinal flora, cleanses intestines |
| **Kidney Stimulation** | birch juice<br>horsetail juice<br>celery juice | birch is a diuretic and eliminates fluids, horsetail strengthens tissues, celery is a diuretic |
| **Laxative** | sauerkraut juice<br>fig syrup | sauerkraut normalizes intestinal flora, stimulates peristaltic movement |
| **Liver Disorders** (functional) | dandelion juice<br>black radish juice<br>nettle juice<br>artichoke juice | dandelion stimulates liver functions, promotes bile flow, black radish relaxes biliary duct, promotes bile flow, nettle purifies, eliminates, artichoke strengthens liver, improves its detoxifying ability |
| **Lumbago** | birch juice<br>celery juice | birch purifies blood, stimulates metabolism, celery is a diuretic and relieves pain in joints |
| **Nervous Irritability** | rosemary juice<br>balm mint juice | effective for nerves and circulation |
| **Nervous Weakness** | St. John's Wort juice<br>oat juice | St. John's Wort juice builds up and oat juice helps the foundation of a strong nervous system |
| **Nervousness** | valerian juice<br>St. John's Wort juice | valerian soothes and calms, St. John's Wort strengthens nervous system |
| **Respiratory Complaints** | coltsfoot juice<br>plantain (ribwort) juice<br>horsetail juice | these juices are cleansing, counteract inflammation, and strengthen the respiratory system |

| When to use | Which Juice(s) | Why |
|---|---|---|
| **Rheumatism** | birch juice<br>nettle juice<br>juniper extract | birch juice and nettle juice act on the metabolism, juniper extract stimulates it |
| **Skin Problems** (blemishes and non-infectious disorders) | nettle juice<br>dandelion juice<br>celery juice | complete treatment with dandelion, nettle and celery juices promotes proper metabolism, dissolves and eliminates waste |
| **Slimming** | nettle juice<br>watercress juice<br>celery juice (taken over a period of time) | powerful diuretics, stimulate elimination |
| **Sore Throats** (from chills) | sage juice<br>camomile juice | sage juice used as a gargle disinfects and cleanses, camomile relieves soreness |
| **Spring Cleansing** and Spring Fatigue | stinging nettle juice<br>plantain juice<br>celery juice | taken over a period of time, these juices activate the metabolism, mobilize toxins and eliminate wastes |
| **Stomach Infections** | garlic juice | adjusts the balance of micro-organisms in the stomach |
| **Stomach and Intestinal Cramps** | silverweed juice<br>wormwood juice | silverweed juice is anti-spasmodic and wormwood juice helps the stomach |
| **Stomach, Low Acidity** | wormwood juice | promotes gastric juice production |
| **Stomach Upsets** | yarrow juice<br>camomile juice | yarrow relieves spasms, camomile soothes and relieves inflammation |
| **Stress Relief** | valerian juice | calms the nerves |
| **Vein and Artery Strengthening** | special plant juice treatment (consisting of yarrow juice, hawthorn juice, bean juice) | yarrow juice improves circulation, hawthorn juice helps the heart and bean juice cleanses, eliminates metabolic waste and strengthens |
| **Wound healing** | echinacea juice | disinfects and promotes healing |

## How To Use Fresh Cellular Plant Juices

The juices will keep indefinitely if left unopened in the original bottle. Once opened they keep six to ten days if stored in a cool place – even longer in the refrigerator. Tinctures, extracts and distillations keep longer than juices once the seal is broken.

As the juices contain all the soluble ingredients of the plant, they are quite concentrated and have a robust flavor. Therefore, it is recommended to dilute them in order to avoid any possible irritations. The only exceptions are fruit juices.

Based on controlled tests and years of experience, the following dosage has been found best: one tablespoon of plant juice diluted in five to six tablespoons of water, tea, milk or soup three times daily. For optimum utilization by the body, take the juice one quarter of an hour before meals or at least five minutes prior to any food consumption.

The dosage can be lowered for wormwood juice. As for hawthorn juice, the dosage can be lowered to one teaspoon diluted, but taken several times daily. Since in such instances one bottle will last more than four to six days, storage in a very cool place is imperative.

What quantity of juice should be taken to effect a complete cure? A definite answer is not possible. It has been pointed out that plant juices act as a therapeutic tool over a certain period of time. This by no means precludes the possibility of improvement after a very short interval; however, even then a continuation over a minimum period of several weeks is recommended to strengthen the beneficial effects.

As far as the vegetable juices are concerned, the period of consumption can be extended indefinitely without any ill effects.

Some juices do bring quick results. These include hawthorn juice for a nervous heart; black radish for a congested gall bladder and liver; and valerian for insomnia or general restlessness. For juices that have a diuretic effect, such as birch, bean and celery as well as juniper extract, one must understand that the elimination of the surplus liquid from the system often only begins after two or three days. The ability of coltsfoot, plantain and horsetail juice to loosen mucus, soothe coughs, reduce inflammation and generally build strength can be hastened as well as increased by mixing the juice with natural, unpasteurized honey.

# III

# Nature's Gifts
# to Mankind

*A cross-section of
medicinal herbs and plants
and their time-proven efficacy
in plant juice therapies*

*"The weed is a plant
whose virtues have not
yet been discovered."*

*Ralph Waldo Emerson*

# Acerola
## *The vitamin C powerhouse*

Is it a berry or is it a cherry? Actually it's both. In the tropics, the acerola is called the "health tree." It is also known as Barbados cherry, West Indian cherry and Puerto Rican cherry, but most commonly as acerola berry. The fruit is native to the West Indies. It was first discovered growing on Puerto Rico, but it is also cultivated and grown on plantations in many tropical regions, especially northern South America and Florida.

The acerola berry resembles a very large cherry - it is about two to four inches in diameter – but instead of one stone it has many tiny seeds. The mature fruit is soft and juicy, with a tart flavor. It is a semi-tropical fruit botanically known as *Malpighia punicifolia*.

Nutritionists value the acerola berry for its high content of natural vitamin C. Scientific investigation has determined that the acerola berry is the richest known source of natural vitamin C, with a single berry packing a generous 85 milligrams. It has been estimated that it would require about 20 kilograms of fresh white cabbage juice to yield as much vitamin C as found in only 20 grams of acerola berries!

The acerola's distinction as a powerhouse of natural vitamin C is unquestionable when compared with other fruits and vegetables rich in vitamin C. The average content of vitamin C per 100 grams is 3,400 mg in acerola juice, 300 mg in rosehip syrup, 200 mg in black currants, 100 mg in green peppers, 80 mg in lemons and 50 mg in orange juice. Besides being the richest source of Vitamin C, acerola also contains significant amounts of minerals, including phosphorus, potassium, calcium and magnesium as well as the pro-vitamin beta-carotene.

The fact that acerola juice is tart in flavor has not added to its popularity as a drink by itself. Like lemon juice, it is most often used as a mixer and to provide vitamin C or flavor. Its fame as the powerhouse of natural vitamin C has obscured another important fact: acerola is very low in calories. With berries weighing in at about two calories each you do not need to worry about your weight when enjoying acerola juice! Use your imagination to prepare some healthy drinks; combine it with hot, mulled apple juice to fight an oncoming cold, or add acerola juice to any medicinal herbal tea.

Although the value of vitamin C has already been established and is documented in numerous medical research reports, its importance to the health of the body is here summarized once more: Vitamin C is required for normal body cell functioning. It is essential to the formation of collagen, bones, teeth, cartilage, skin and capillary walls, and promotes the formation of strong connective tissue. It also helps build resistance to respiratory ailments, such as the common cold.

In the official U.S. Government publication *Food, Yearbook of Agriculture*, Dr. Mary L. Dodds says: "Anemia has been associated with a lack of vitamin C. The dietary abuse that results in a lack of vitamin C is likely to produce other deficiencies."

Vitamin C has been recognized by Nobel laureate Dr. Prof. Linus Pauling and other scientists, as an important antioxidant in the prevention and treatment of cancer. Since the body neither makes nor stores vitamin C, it must be continually replenished through food and nutritional supplements, for which acerola juice remains the best natural choice.

*As a man thinketh
in his heart, so is he.*

*Anonymous*

# Artichoke
## *A natural liver tonic*

The artichoke (*Cynara scolymus*) belongs to the thistle family. While the size of the flower heads is the most valued and sought after feature in commercial cultivation of the artichoke, the plant's leaves are of equal importance for medicinal purposes. Active ingredients include the bitter substance *cynarin*, fatty acids, enzymes and vitamins.

The artichoke thrives best in a warm climate. It is mostly encountered in Mediterranean regions where it not only grows wild but is commercially cultivated. The plant juice, obtained from fresh-pressed flower heads and leaves, is a perfect example of the old saying "May your food be your medicine."

To discover the medicinal uses of this plant juice, Walther Schoenenberger combined ancient knowledge (2,000 years ago artichokes were considered food only the rich could afford) with the latest scientific research of the cells and their biochemical actions. From this he obtained new concepts and insights regarding the elements of fresh artichokes: they are extremely beneficial to the liver.

Pure natural juice pressed from flower heads and leaves will intensify the action of the liver by promoting the build-up of protein throughout the whole body. Thus, the liver's essential function – to eliminate toxins from the blood – is favorably influenced. In this way, the action of pure artichoke juice contributes to the general well-being of the whole system.

Pure artichoke juice is a natural biological remedy, ideal for therapies or treatments where the constitution of the liver needs to be regenerated. Hand-in-hand with such a liver-purifying, liver-protecting process, old age symptoms – which usually originate with deteriorating liver tissues – are delayed in quite a natural way. Liver disorders are often manifested in symptoms such as flatulence, nausea, migraine headaches, diarrhea or constipation.

In addition to stimulating the production and flow of bile, artichoke juice has a similar effect on the function of the kidneys and strengthens the metabolic assimilation of fats. And last, but not least, the cholesterol level of the blood is reduced.

Such a beneficial stimulation and purification of the vital liver functions by artichoke therapy usually results in an increased feeling of well-being and a new-found zest for life. It has been said, and quite rightly so, that "the condition of the liver depends on how the *liver* treats the liver."

When combined with fresh-pressed cellular watercress juice, the effects of artichoke juice are greatly enhanced.

Because of all the above-mentioned beneficial properties, artichoke juice may be combined for a synergistic effect with nettle, potato and tomato juices to cleanse the body most effectively and to lose weight naturally and safely.

*See: Regenerative Therapy; Slimming/Weight Reducing Therapy*

# Asparagus
## *The weight loss gourmet*

Asparagus (*Liliaceae* or *Asparagus officinalis*) is cultivated on a large scale as a gourmet vegetable. But it is seldom used for medicinal purposes anymore, even though its medicinal applications can be traced back thousands of years to China. In ancient Greece, the physician Dioscorides prescribed asparagus to stimulate and strengthen kidney functions, while Hippocrates, the father of medicine, gave it to his overweight patients and to all with blemished skin.

The historical use of asparagus as a home remedy has been well documented for kidney and bladder complaints, dropsy, for supporting liver functions, as well as for relieving rheumatism and gout.

The woody root stock of asparagus is grounded deep below the surface. Early in spring, white, finger-thick shoots sprout to the surface. Asparagus stems grow up to one meter long with small, thin leaves and white blossoms which turn into small red berries. These berries can be dried and ground into a coffee substitute. Only the root and the young shoots are medicinally valuable.

The active ingredients in asparagus are: asparagine (an acid), arginin, asparagose, chelindonic acid, coniferin (a glycocide), choline, saponines, flavonoids and a vast number of minerals, most significantly potassium, as well as trace elements. All these substances act together to accelerate the metabolism –

fat cells get rid of excess metabolic waste, liver functions are stimulated, and the kidney and bladder get a kickstart to expel more water. Asparagine as an ingredient of asparagus is of uttermost importance for a healthy cell structure and cell renewal.

Asparagus is a dream come true for all those who are overweight and want to lose weight without going hungry. Though one would not talk about an "asparagus diet," it is a new and safe way to support a calorie-reduced diet for shedding some pounds. By changing to a primarily vegetarian or a lacto-ovo vegetarian diet supported by asparagus juice you can loose about eight pounds in two weeks.

Nature has certainly provided foods throughout the seasons when they are most beneficial for us. After a long winter our bodies may become sluggish, slightly overweight and loaded with toxins – it is time for house cleaning! Asparagus lends itself wonderfully to the task. For a two week diet you need about ³/₄ litre asparagus juice, or four bottles if you buy the juice from a health food store. Take two tablespoons of juice in the morning and in the evening, diluted in a glass of water.

*For diet suggestions see: Slimming/Weight Reducing Therapy*

## Balm Mint or Melissa
### *A most beloved and versatile home remedy*

Nature has provided us with both stimulating and calming substances, hiding them in all kinds of wild plants scattered over all the earth. We do not know just how mankind first became aware of particular plants and their proper uses. However, it is certain that the highly aromatic plants were especially conspicuous, inviting their use as drink, nourishment and medication. Small wonder then, that the strongly scented lemon balm mint (*Melissa officinalis*) attracted attention very early. It is common in the Mediterranean area and in the Near East, but it is also naturalized in some places in the United States. It is now cultivated mainly as a culinary herb, but it still grows wild, flowering in July and August in fields, gardens and along the roadsides. Due to its etheric oils, of which *citral* and *citronella* are the most pronounced, the whole plant smells like lemon when bruised. Other active ingredients include tannin, resin, bitters and minerals.

Balm mint belongs to the *Labiate* plants, a plant family with many aromatic representatives. Found centuries ago in peasant gardens, its medicinal strength was quickly recognized and handed down in old herbal books.

Balm juice is a remedy for common female complaints, for all sorts of nervous problems, and for hysteria, melancholy, flatulence, colic, chronic bronchial catarrh and some forms of asthma. Further indications are for migraines, toothaches and, during pregnancy, for headaches and dizziness. It is also prescribed in cases of nervous heart disorders.

Schoenenberger's fresh-pressed cellular balm mint juice is free from alcohol and has a mild flavor and aroma. Take one tablespoon three times daily before meals (for sensitive constitutions and children take one teaspoon) diluted with camomile tea or water. The effectiveness of balm mint is increased when taken as a therapy course over six weeks.

*Take balm for her pain,*
*if so she may be healed.*

*Bible, King James Version*
*Jeremiah 51:8*

# Bean
## *A rare combination of effective ingredients*

Nutritional research over the past few decades has impressively shown to what extent health is related to the food we eat. A balanced diet is essential for the supply of necessary proteins, starches, essential fatty acids, vitamins, minerals and other trace elements, all of which contribute to "feeling in the best of health."

There are many ordinary vegetables, plants and herbs that, due to some specific ingredient, could also be classified as medicinal. The potato, for instance, in its pure substance, has a definite influence on the rhythmic functioning of the heart.

In this same context, we find the lowly string bean *(Phaseolus vulgaris)*. It is a wonderful combination of many effective ingredients, such as proteins, rich supplies of silicium dioxide (which improves skin conditions and is diuretic), trace elements of choline (which stimulate the liver's metabolism), potassium, manganese, sulphur, chlorine, phosphorus, lime, magnesium, iron, aluminum, cobalt, nickel and silica.

The bean's extraordinary diuretic properties are mainly due to its high mineral content and its ability to stimulate the kidneys. However, in cases of heart and circulatory weaknesses, bean juice should only be used where no organic damage exists.

The extraordinary importance of plant and fruit nourishment can be realized in the string bean's potential to assist diabetics. The string bean stabilizes blood sugar, thus fresh-pressed bean juice is a natural substitute for insulin.

Fresh-pressed bean juice is the only way to get all the soluble ingredients of the bean in its natural and concentrated form. Only the fresh juice avoids any reduction or changes of the vegetable's original medicinal properties, particularly the organic ones.

As diabetics are now able to monitor blood sugar levels themselves, they will discover the positive effect of string bean juice within a short while after regular use.

# Birch
## *The "blood" of the tree*

The cellular juices of the birch leaves (*Betula alba*) are rich in a great many components of the highest quality, especially in springtime, since that is when they contain the necessary ingredients for the new growth and maintenance of the tree itself. In addition, there are freshly produced organic substances in the rising sap, such as the yellow pigmentation, the sugars and resin. Over 30 ingredients are known to us, including etheric oils, flavonoids, resins, tannin and numerous minerals. Further research with new methods is expected to yield deeper insight into the complex structure of birch sap.

The birch tree is one of the oldest tree species gracing the landscapes of western and central Europe and North America. Its healing qualities have been known since ancient times and the birch tree plays an important role in both folklore and folk medicine. The sap, providing it is natural and not fermented, is medicinally most valuable as a diuretic.

Today's natural healing methods also recognize the great importance of fresh birch leaf juice for the strengthening and stimulation of the kidneys and the bladder. This includes cases of light catarrh in these organs, provided there are no symptoms of severe organic deficiencies. Furthermore, the action of birch juice reduces the protein content of the urine.

In addition to the above, birch juice is used as a diuretic remedy in cases of rheumatic and arthritis complaints. It exerts a curative influence on such symptoms as muscular pains and swelling of the joints. To obtain an enduring effect, dietary changes should also be initiated during the treatment, particularly the complete elimination of all uric-acid-forming foods, especially meat. In such cases, it is advisable to consult a nutrition-oriented physician.

Birch juice has two essential functions:

1. It improves and strengthens the renal system. This is beneficially supported by the secondary effect of reducing the protein content of the urine.

2. It significantly promotes the elimination of uric acid. Remember, the concentration of uric acid in our blood is considered the cause of painful arthritis, of some rheumatic complaints and of gout – all of them widespread diseases of our civilization!

Its best known folk use is to promote hair growth, but folk medicine has several other uses for birch juice and fresh birch-leaf tea, such as a mild sedative or for bathing.

*See: Arthritis and Rheumatism Therapy; Kidney and Bladder Disorders Therapy*

# Black Radish
## *Brings new life to both liver and gallbladder*

Although its ancestry and place in the plant system is still under debate, it is a historic fact that black radish (*Raphanus sativus*) is a cultivated plant of considerable age. The pharaohs of Egypt had this plant depicted on the walls of their sepulchral chambers. The Greek writer Herodotus mentions this fact in one of his books, and the Roman Plinius left documentation about its healing properties. Black radish is also included in the famous *Capitulare* of Charles the Great (800 AD). This plant's applications and recipes were handed down through medieval herbal books right into modern medicine.

Today, black radish still enjoys great esteem as a medicinal plant. It has been proven that fresh black radish juice contains certain ingredients of great importance for the formation and the unobstructed flow of bile. Thus, not only does it prevent congestion of bile, but it also avoids inflammation of the gallbladder or formation of gallstones. However, should such congestion or inflammation of the bile ducts or stones already exist, black radish juice, used over a period of time in a therapeutic approach, produces results so striking that present-day biochemists did laboratory tests to isolate the ingredients. They came to the conclusion that, from the chemical point of view, the major healing benefits stem from the sulphuric etheric oil, called *raphanol*, a glycoside, as well as an ingredient similar to mustard oil and various minerals.

Black radish juice also has a mild laxative effect. When combined with honey, this juice is soothing in cases of obstinate coughs caused by chills, since it assists in elimination of congestive mucus.

For strengthening the liver and in cases of bilious complaints, a combination of black radish juice and dandelion juice has shown best results when taken under the regimen of a therapy lasting at least three weeks, in conjunction with a low fat, vegetarian diet.

*See: Liver and Gallbladder Therapy*

# Borage
## *Increases your joy in living*

It seems strange that ancient wisdom about the favorable influence of borage juice (*Borago officinalis*) on depression, melancholy and nerve conditions finds so little application in our time. We seem to prefer the use of alcohol and pep pills.

The old Romans certainly knew the wonderful effects of borage juice for alleviating depression and hypochondria. *"Ego borago, gaudia semper ago,"* meaning "I, borage, always bring joy," was a well-known quote. Medieval herbal books lauded borage for its strengthening qualities for both heart and brain (mind) and for its ability to "re-awaken the melancholy to gladness and pleasurable delights." At the same time its ability to purify the blood and reduce feverishness was widely recognized. The synergistic effect of the active ingredients of hormone-like substances, mucilage, tannins, resin, silica, etheric oils, and minerals is mildly laxative and diuretic.

This old lore has lately been confirmed in our new "scientific" herbal books. The appreciation of the beneficial influence of borage juice on the state of the mind – that is the psychological rather than the physical – has been renewed. Our modern psychiatry is recognizing more and more how closely both our mental and spiritual well-being are connected with our bodies. Upon re-examining the causes of depression, for instance, it was found that poor circulation, or some toxicity in the system, was often responsible. Extensive investigations are now underway to search for the special elements in the borage plant that act so beneficially on the capillaries. We already know of the strong blood-purifying properties of borage juice which, at least partly, explain its stimulating effect on the nervous system and brain.

The pressed juice of fresh borage plants is, first of all, suggested as a remedy for melancholy – keeping in mind that it stimulates, energizes and renews the zest for life. It is the most natural anti-depressant there is.

Though borage is a widespread kitchen and medicinal herb, only the fresh plant is useful, not the dried herb. Drying this high water content plant is problematic – most of its aroma and medicinal ingredients are destroyed in the process. Fortunately borage is easy to grow. Many gardens are decorated with this annual and most nurseries carry it in the herb section. Once planted it will flourish abundantly until frost sets in. For juicing, pick the upper one third of the plant, leaves and blue blossoms. Using an electric juicer a hand held bunch of borage will yield enough juice to last a few days.

*See: Female Complaints Therapy*

# Camomile
## *The "wonder drug" of nature*

If you wander through flowering meadows in southern Europe during June or July, you are sure to find the sweet smelling camomile (*Matricaria chamomilla*) growing wild. Similarly, you'll see it as a cultivated plant in many gardens.

For centuries, camomile tea has been a home remedy for nervous conditions: insomnia, neuralgia, lumbago, rheumatic problems and skin rashes. It also tends to reduce inflammation and to facilitate bowel movement without acting directly as a purgative.

Unlike herbal tea, fresh camomile juice combines *all* the properties of the living plant, and these manifold components act on the human body in a beneficial and relaxing way. Besides the blue healing oil *azulene*, valued mainly for its soothing qualities, camomile juice contains a number of active substances, such as bitters, flavonoids, linoleic acid, choline, salicylic acid, a glycoside and minerals. Foremost is its influence on the nerves, as it relieves spasms and tensions, irritability and hyper-sensitivity. It is equally efficacious for toothaches, cramps and gallstone colics. Camomile juice is also used in cases of stomach-aches, nervous cramps, flatulence and inflammation of mucus membranes of the gastro-intestinal system.

In order to achieve a complete restoration of the body, the juice should be taken for an extended period of up to two months. However, on principle, all inflammatory symptoms should be treated by a physician first. A diet low in salt and supplemented with vitamins B and C (preferably through vegetables, wholemeal bread and acerola juice) would greatly assist the therapeutic approach.

*Let nature have her way.*
*She knows her business better than we do.*

*Montaigne*

# Carrot
## *The all-round vegetable*

The carrot (*Daucus carota*) is one of the few cultivated vegetables that has descended from a wild-growing indigenous plant. This annual or biennial plant can still be found wild throughout farmlands, pastures and meadows, but this variety, known under the common names of bee's-nest plant, bird's-nest root or Queen Anne's lace, has a tough, white *inedible* root.

In Roman times, carrots were imported from the Germanic tribes, and Emperor Tiberius was quite partial to them. Charles the Great of France had special areas in his kitchen gardens allotted for the carrot, and he issued specific instructions regarding its proper cultivation. In thirteenth century herbal books we find the carrot listed as a medicinal plant. Until the potato was imported from America, this root was the staple food of rich and poor alike.

Raw carrots contain nearly all the minerals and vitamins required by the human body. They are an exceedingly rich source of vitamin A in its precursor form, beta-carotene, and of enzymes and glucose. Carrots are also a fair source of vitamins B and C. In recent years carrots have been recognized as one of the most valuable vegetables, perhaps the best balanced from the standpoint of vitamins and minerals. Scientists tell us that the iron and calcium in carrots is almost entirely assimilated by the human body. Carrots also contain potassium, magnesium and manganese, as well as ample proportions of the strong cleansing elements sulphur, chlorine and phosphorus.

It is no wonder then, that fresh carrot juice is an effective remedy for diarrhea and is easily digestible for those suffering from stomach and intestinal problems. Carrot juice is also useful for preventing putrefaction in the intestines and for gastro-intestinal catarrh. Its content of potassium salts accounts for the diuretic action. It also contains an essential oil that is effective against ringworms. (Just eat two to three raw carrots a day for several days.) It is often recommended to take carrot juice for stomach acidity and heartburn, and of course, everyone knows that carrots are good for the eyes, due to vitamin A in the carotene. This vitamin is important for proper vision, especially night vision.

Carrot juice was successfully applied in the "pre-vitamin era" for chronic bronchitis and infectious diseases, but it proved most strikingly effective in cases of malnutrition in babies and infants. Because of its concentration of nourishing vitamins and minerals, carrot juice (particularly since it excludes all fibrous roughage) can be tolerated as a supplementary feeding even by babies a few months old.

As a tonic and restorative, fresh carrot juice is well matched with spinach juice.

# Celery
## *An excellent dietary remedy*

Celery (*Apium graveolus*) is a widely cultivated, biennial plant which also grows wild in salty soils of North and South America, Europe and Africa. Thus, celery is known and valued practically all over the world. It is used as an appetizer to improve the taste of other dishes, to stimulate digestion, as well as to eliminate excessive fluids from the body. All this was known to the ancient cultures. Hippocrates used celery in treatments over 2,400 years ago!

Present in celery are a number of noteworthy elements which have aroused considerable medical interest. Today, nutritionists advise the use of every part of the plant as a beneficial food. The stalk contains 93.7 percent pure, unpolluted water and is rich in calcium, sodium, potassium, phosphorus and iron. Celeriac, the knob-like root, is a source of potassium, sodium, calcium, iron, silicon, much vitamin B and some A. Since the celery juice is obtained from the fresh green leaves and from the fresh celeriac of the plant, it consequently combines the so-called "reserve powers" of celeriac with the vital elements formed by the chlorophyll of the green leaves. Here we find a wealth of chloride minerals combined with alkaline ash, something the body greatly needs.

These same elements (already known for centuries) exert their beneficial action on certain diseases. First of all, celery juice is appreciated for its stimulating effect on digestion as a diuretic, and for its general dissolving and discharging action of waste materials, mainly through the kidneys.

In this natural way, celery juice helps the organism to rid itself of accumulated metabolic waste. This has a favorable effect on all symptoms and complaints, such as rheumatism and arthritis caused by such accumulations. As well, it is a tonic and restorative for the nervous and glandular systems, and is equally helpful for flatulence, chronic pulmonary catarrh, tendencies toward overweight and lack of appetite. Celery also promotes the onset of menstruation.

*See: Blood Purifying Therapy; Slimming/Weight Reducing Therapy*

## Coltsfoot
### *Relieves asthma, bronchial catarrh, cough and loosens phlegm*

Coltsfoot is one of the time-tested remedies for respiratory problems. In the time of Hippocrates, coltsfoot (*Tussilago farafara*) was used in cases of debilitating chronic chest illnesses, such as bronchitis and asthma. The Greek doctor Dioscorides favored it for chest complaints in general. Old folklore agreed with the ancients and, right up until the sixteenth century, coltsfoot was applied for all persistent problems affecting the lungs.

Present-day natural therapy carries on with the tradition set by previous medical knowledge, and coltsfoot is used for hoarseness and the loosening of phlegm as well as cases of chronic bronchitis and enlarged bronchi. The general indications for the medical use of coltsfoot are the various types of catarrhs of the lungs and of the bronchi, and for loosening of mucus. For strengthening general bodily resistance, but especially the resistance of the respiratory tract against colds or flu, coltsfoot is most beneficial when combined with rosehip juice.

Chemical analysis of this plant shows an extraordinarily high content of minerals (17 percent), some tannic acid, bitters, etheric oils and proteins. When it is burned, the ashes contain potassium, sulphur and silica. The powerfully effective expectorant qualities of coltsfoot are mainly due to its nitric salts, which also support mucus secretion and alleviate fever.

It is most interesting to note that the use of fresh-pressed juice is recommended in the ancient medical history of coltsfoot. The old texts say the juice is the best medium to retain all of the plant's ingredients and preserve them in a complete and natural form.

Coltsfoot juice can be tolerated even by children, and it is best taken hourly or several times a day, diluted in a proportion of six to one in hot milk or hot water with honey. A most beneficial effect is achieved when combined with plantain (ribwort) juice as a therapeutic approach for the above-listed ailments.

*See: Respiratory Tract Therapy*

# Dandelion
## *The incredible edible*

Although the virtues of the dandelion (*Taraxacum officinale*) have been appreciated since the distant past, today it is mostly ignored or looked upon as a weed that must be eliminated. The name comes from the French *dent de lion*, meaning "lion's tooth," which refers to the saw-edged leaves of the plant. Related to the sunflower or aster family, dandelions are known as blow balls, puff balls as well as heart fever grass, wild endive and *pushki* by the Russians. The Latin name *Taraxacum officinale*, again refers to the tooth-edged leaf of the "lion." The "official" part of the plant is its sturdy root, which is often a component in prescriptions and is known as *Taraxacum*, a bitter substance. J. I. Lighthall, a North American Indian medicine man from Kansas writes about dandelion: "This is a plant that should never be dried. We know by experience that it loses its medical properties when dried, consequently, the green and the roots are parts in demand for medicinal virtue."

Most species of dandelion originated in Europe or Asia, but it now flourishes in all cool and temperate zones of the world, almost throughout the year. According to ancient lore and experience, dandelion is helpful as a bitter tonic and a laxative, valued for the heart and liver, gallstones, spleen, rheumatism, gastric headaches, dyspepsia, indigestion, dropsy or urinary complaints, diabetes, typhoid fever, night

---

[1] J. I. Lighthall, *Indian Household Medicine Guide*, Peoria, Ill:1883.

sweats, inflammation of the bowels, fever and debility. Quite a roster for such a "weed"! It was also thought to be very helpful to the female organs and beneficial for problems of the skin – even freckles. An old gypsy and Indian remedy for removing warts or corns is to apply the milk from a broken dandelion stem two or three times a day, letting it dry each time on the skin. This cure was believed to be both rapid and effective.

So much for old folklore and popular use of this famous weed. What about today's scientific opinion? Would it surprise you to know that the ancient claims have been confirmed? It has been found true that dandelion stimulates the flow of bile and function of the liver.

Dandelion is, of course, edible in its raw form, as a salad, provided the young tender leaves are gathered before the plant has bloomed. That is when they are more nutritious, contain all the oils and healing ingredients and are not yet bitter. But the ideal way to take this most versatile plant is in the liquid form all year round – as a fresh-pressed plant juice. In this way you get all the components intact in their natural proportion, minus the roughage – a form most acceptable to a sensitive or greatly debilitated organism.

Dandelion juice is truly a natural stimulant for the liver to produce more free-flowing bile. On the whole, the general well-being induced by taking this juice is due to the stimulation of the entire metabolism as well as the liver cells. This is achieved through the wealth of minerals contained in the plant, such as potassium, calcium, manganese, sodium, silica, sulphur, phosphorus and many more.

Dandelion has two particularly important uses today: to promote the formation of bile and to remove excess water from the body in conditions resulting from liver problems. The root especially affects all forms of secretion and excretion from the body and, by serving to remove poison from the body, it acts as a tonic and stimulant as well. The fresh-pressed juice is considered the most effective way of taking the root.

For chronic rheumatism, gout and stiff joints, it is best to follow an eight-week dandelion therapy, in combination with nettle juice and celery juice. If dandelion juice is combined with black radish juice as therapy for bilious and liver complaints, it will bring about the desired results.

*See: Blood Purifying Therapy*

# Echinacea
## *The immune system booster*

The Sioux Indians of North America have extremely good knowledge of the medicinal properties of echinacea – commonly called Purple Coneflower. Besides applying this herb as a first aid for snake bites, the Indians scraped the fresh root and used it for treating blood poisoning, infectious conditions and hydrophobia. In North America, echinacea *(Echinacea angustifolia)* has a long folk medicine history of killing bacteria (antiseptic), promoting wound healing (alterative) and inhibiting inflammation. It is also effective in the treatment of diseases due to blood impurities, for example, boils, abscesses and carbuncles. Even treatment of acne with echinacea has been recorded.

There are two different species of echinacea that the Indians regard as sacred: *Echinacea purpurea* and *E. angustifolia*. The latter of the two varieties has a deep penetrating tap root, while purpurea's root is more shallow. From a medicinal point of view both are of equal value.

Echinacea is native to the prairie regions of North America, west of Ohio. This common perennial plant with beautiful blooms is a popular medicinal herb on this continent, but only recently has it come to be appreciated in Europe. It only occurred there as a rare, cultivated plant until this century, when it was introduced to Dr. Alfred Vogel by Black Eagle, a tribal chief in South Dakota. Dr. Vogel recognized immediately the potential healing power of the plant, and started cultivating echinacea as a medicinal herb in Switzerland.

Echinacea has stimulated keen interest among modern researchers who have worked to isolate the active ingredients. What they found, other than volatile oils and resin, were two polysacharide components, inulin and echinasin, which, as they discovered, have the ability to reinforce the body's own defense mechanisms. Medical science began to realize that echinacea was a very remarkable plant indeed! The two polysacharides are primarily responsible for the immunostimulatory activities of echinacea. These actions make it especially effective in fighting viral infections and, to an even greater extent, cancerous conditions.

A properly functioning immune system is vital; without a good defense mechanism we could not survive. As the immune system is weakened by our unnatural, modern way of life it is good to know that echinacea juice as a herbal remedy can play an important role in keeping us healthy. Echinacea activates and strengthens the immune system and is therefore a tremendous aid in increasing the body's resistance to micro-organisms and all infections – viral, fungal as well as bacterial. It also strengthens the lymphatic system, and it helps those who suffer constant attacks of colds and catarrh.

With the first sign of an oncoming illness a tablespoon of echinacea juice is recommended. Take four to five times daily, as long as the condition persists. Echinacea, like any other herbal remedy, should be discontinued once health has been restored.

# Fennel
## *A delightfully aromatic spice and medicinal herb*

This perennial, lacy-looking plant grows wild in the Mediterranean area and in Asia Minor, but is commonly cultivated in North America and Europe.

Scarcely any other plant has as many uses as fennel – as a medicinal, a vegetable and a flavoring. Fennel (*Foeniculum vulgare*) belongs to the group of herbs whose umbelliferous blossoms contain a typical aromatic oil. In the past, the medicinal parts were considered to be the root and the seed only. Now fennel juice is pressed from those green parts of the plant growing above the ground and has the typical odor of licorice. These aromatic, etheric substances not only stimulate our tastebuds and possibly the sense of smell, but deeply affect the whole organism. One of their special characteristics, the ability to dissolve fat and protein-fat layers, provides evidence of their many-sided effectiveness.

Pure-plant fennel juice soothes the stomach nerves and is an effective remedy for flatulence and abdominal cramps. It can be used successfully against colds for loosening and expelling mucus. Fennel is also quite effective for coughs, hoarseness and chest catarrhs. Nursing mothers ought to take fennel juice to ensure sufficient milk supply. Fennel soothes stomach-aches and relieves flatulence. Children love fennel juice.

# Fig Syrup
## *A truly "fruity" natural laxative*

The fig tree (*Ficus carica*) grows in profusion in its native Mediterranean region and is cultivated elsewhere for its fruit.

The fleshy, pear-shaped fruit we call the fig (it is botanically known as the *syconium*) varies in color from greenish-yellow to purple, depending on the variety. Ripe figs have an almost honey-sweet flavor and are most tasty when eaten fresh.

The fig has mildly laxative properties and is often used in combination with senna and carminative herbs. When you have a cold, a concoction of figs acts as a demulcent to soothe the mucus membranes of the respiratory passage.

Fig syrup does not contain any chemical mixtures. It is a mild and quite delicious remedy that helps to normalize the action of the bowels, thereby preventing constipation.

# Garlic
## *The classsic medicine*

Garlic (*Allium sativum*), which hails from the Orient, is one of our most important remedies. It belongs to the family of lilies (*Liliaceae*) and is related to the onion. Both are known for their pungent odor because of their specific sulphuric etheric oils.

Tracing the history of civilization, it is very interesting to note that garlic was at first a "tool of magic power" in the hands of the physician-priest or medicine man. Only gradually did its spell-binding nimbus in the art of exorcism die out. Today this strong-smelling bulb has established itself as a most valuable medicinal remedy in every household.

Hippocrates regarded garlic highly. Odysseus used it to counteract Circe's charm. In Virgil's *Idylls* its efficiency against snake bites is pointed out. To the slaves building the pyramids, garlic was a supplier of strength and staying power. The soldiers of medieval times swore that it increased their courage, and in the older *Edda* version, garlic is mentioned as a fortifying and protecting medicinal plant. The *Talmud* lauds it as a satisfying food which warms the body, lifts the spirits and sustains cheerfulness.

Garlic's outstanding quality is its ability to stimulate the activity of the digestive organs and therefore relieve various problems associated with poor digestion. As an expectorant, it is useful for chronic stomach and intestinal catarrh as well as for chronic bronchitis. Garlic also regulates the action of the liver and the gallbladder. It is helpful for all intestinal infections, such as dysentery, cholera, typhoid fever and for problems caused by putrefactive intestinal bacteria. A tincture of garlic lowers blood pressure and helps to counteract arteriosclerosis.

Garlic is especially convincing in its action on the vascular system because it dilates and relaxes the capillary blood vessels. Its beneficial effect on blood circulation and heart action can bring relief for many common bodily complaints.

Garlic juice diluted (one teaspoon to one-half litre of water) can be used as an enema for intestinal worms, particularly pinworms.

In order to avoid habituation, garlic juice therapies should take only four weeks. Such therapy is the ideal remedy for arteriosclerosis, both as prophylaxis and as treatment. The symptoms of this disease, such as headache and buzzing in the ears, are favorably influenced by garlic juice.

Walther Schoenenberger succeeded in developing a unique, stabilized garlic juice in which the odor is minimal, since it contains the effective etheric oils in a "plant-bound" form, as it is in the unbroken garlic bud.

The effects of Schoenenberger's stabilized garlic juice can be summarized as follows:

1. It efficiently supports the function of the body in geriatric cases, beneficially affecting heart and circulation, hypertension (in milder instances), a tendency towards headaches and low resistance to disease.

2. As part of a therapeutic approach, garlic juice can be combined with ramson, hawthorn or mistletoe juices to ease the discomfort of arteriosclerosis.

*See: Arteriosclerosis Therapy*

# Hawthorn
## *A heart tonic*

The last few decades have brought hawthorn (*Crataegus oxyacantha*) to the top of the "bestseller list" in natural medications. This phenomenon is singularly tied to the rise in cardiovascular disease, one of the major killers among men, and not only those in their 50s and 60s but nowadays even from their late 30s. Once it was believed that the general pressures of living and competing were the root of this type of heart problem – today we know that a diet rich in saturated and hydrogenated fats (trans fatty acids) is the cause of cardiovascular disease.[1] Recently, natural therapists have rediscovered the beneficial effects of hawthorn juice on the functions of the heart and the circulation in general.

We need not wonder why this plant has been singled out for helping the cardiovascular system when we learn about its properties and varied uses as an anti-spasmodic, cardiac, sedative and vasodilatory. In plain language, this means that hawthorn juice is a special biological remedy for treatment of the heart. It not only relaxes muscular tensions, but it also stimulates the flow of blood to the heart, thereby improving the metabolic condition of the cardiac muscles. Because hawthorn widens the coronary blood vessels, it promotes an increased intake of oxygen. Hand-in-hand with this is a normalization of blood pressure.

---

[1] Erasmus, Udo., *Fats that Heal – Fats that Kill*, 1993.

Hawthorn juice, obtained from the leaves and blossoms of the plant, is also indicated for the soothing of the "highly taxed heart" in the overweight, laborers and athletes; for the prevention of overstrain; and for convalescents, particularly after infectious diseases. It has also proven very beneficial in cases of arteriosclerosis.

When combined with garlic juice, hawthorn juice will lower blood pressure even more, and reduce stress on the circulatory system. When celery juice is added to this mixture, the diuretic effect will relieve the work of the heart by eliminating surplus fluids from the system. For best results, these therapies should go hand-in-hand with a proper diet.

While hawthorn juice can be taken without hesitation and without danger over an extended period of time, the same rule applies as with all heart conditions: do nothing without consulting your own nutrition-oriented physician, naturopath or herbal practitioner.

*See: Arteriosclerosis Therapy; Heart and Circulation Therapy, Regenerative Therapy*

# Horseradish
## *A natural antibiotic*

The medicinal part of the horseradish (*Armoracia lapathifolia*) is the root or rhizome, known to us by its strong odor and pungent taste. It is very popular as a piquant spice to enhance the wholesomeness of many foods. The desire arose to find a way of preserving the valuable ingredients and etheric oils of the rhizome to benefit health the whole year round. However, since the woody root did not lend itself to a liquefying process, Walther Schoenenberger solved the problem by making a distillate. To date, Schoenenberger's horseradish distillate remains the only product of its kind in the marketplace.

This distillate exerts a strong effect on all mucus membranes, which explains its extraordinary stimulation of the digestive system and general body metabolism. After a period of time, horseradish distillate strengthens the peristaltic action of the intestines and flatulence is completely eliminated. This indicates an intensification of circulation prompted by the action of the horseradish etheric oils. For this reason horseradish distillate is used externally for rheumatism; when the affected area is rubbed with the distillate, the blood flow is stimulated and pain eased. Similarly, these oils stimulate and dilate the capillary system, thus fostering better blood and lymph circulation, and this, in turn, improves kidney, liver, gallbladder and pancreas function. This also explains why horseradish distillate stimulates the appetite and digestion, especially after eating rich foods.

Horseradish distillate is recommended in therapies for rheumatic complaints (due to its diuretic effect) and stimulation of the metabolism. For alleviating catarrhs, coughs and asthma, diluted horseradish distillate combined with honey is often recommended. It is interesting to note that after taking horseradish distillate, or eating it fresh with meals, the feeling of thirst is reduced.

In recent clinical tests, researchers confirmed a strong antibiotic quality in horseradish that reduces fever and inflammation. In a further analysis, a substance was found called *sinigrin* from which the horseradish oil is derived through a biological process. The main components of the oil are those of the sulphuric mustard oils.

In summary, horseradish distillate stimulates the appetite and the digestive tract. It is a strong diuretic and improves blood circulation, thus it is most beneficial for treatment of rheumatic, arthritic and/or gout complaints. Honey-diluted horseradish distillate is recommended for alleviating catarrhs, coughs and asthma.

*See: Arthritis and Rheumatism Therapy*

# Horsetail (Shave Grass)
## *A natural diuretic*

One hundred and fifty years ago the famous Father Sebastian Kneipp revived the popularity of this herbal "drug," and in the 1980s Maria Treben resurrected its popular usage. Although its value seems unknown to orthodox medicine, horsetail (*Esquisetum arvense*) was recognized for its potent diuretic and astringent qualities in the eighteenth century. It was used by Dioscorides in ancient Greece, and found its way into medieval herb books via Plinius and Albertus Magnus. Folklore had many uses for this wild plant. Horsetail has proven useful in lung problems, including TB (its silica content is said to stabilize scar tissue). The juice of the plant – essentially the sterile stem – is good for anemia created by internal bleeding from stomach ulcers, since it promotes blood clotting.

Apart from being an excellent tonic for the sensitive pulmonary tissues, horsetail juice also strengthens the body's defenses while purifying at the same time. This is due to the silica which increases the amount of white blood corpuscles. It is particularly beneficial in cases of inflammation of the skin, mucus membranes, and other tissues, and because of its diuretic property, is recommended for all complaints of the urinary tract, including inflammation of the bladder.

Natural fresh-pressed cellular juice of the horsetail plant is recommended for all respiratory problems. Combined with plantain (ribwort) juice, it alleviates bronchial catarrhs and especially chronic bronchitis. As a complete therapeutic approach, the addition of coltsfoot juice to the previously mentioned juices is most beneficial since it loosens phlegm and cleanses the affected organs.

*See: Kidney and Bladder Disorders Therapy; Respiratory Tract Therapy*

*A healthy mind and spirit*
*dwell in a healthy body.*

*Anonymous*

# Juniper
## *A natural antiseptic*

This evergreen shrub grows up to 25 feet tall under favorable circumstances, and is found from the Arctic circle to the southernmost countries of Europe, Asia and America. The medicinal parts are the deep blue berries and new twigs.

Juniper (*Juniperus oxycedrus*) was highly recommended by Hippocrates and Paracelsus and, in medieval times, the twigs were used to fumigate sick rooms. Later the berries were taken internally because of their alleged antiseptic qualities derived from the etheric oils.

The berries contain several types of sugars (glucose, grape sugar), some fatty acids, enzymes, wax, resin, organic acids, a bitter ingredient called *juniperin* and numerous minerals.

The most important component for medicinal application of the juniper extract is certainly the etheric oil. It has a refreshing odor, is a strong germicide and stimulates blood circulation and kidney functions, acting as a diuretic and a natural remedy for rheumatic complaints.

Juniper extract is appreciated as a restorative and is indicated for blood purification. The *juniperin* stimulates digestion, and can help overcome a lack of appetite, gastric problems or tendencies to flatulence. No wonder then, that juniper extract is an ideal remedy to be incorporated in all springtime cleansing and blood purification therapies.

**Caution:** Juniper extract should not be taken when kidney inflammation exists. It should not be used during pregnancy.

*Our bodies are our garden,*
*to which our wills are gardeners.*

*William Shakespeare*

# Mistletoe
## *A benefactor to your circulation*

Both the American mistletoe (*Phoradendron flavescens*) and the European mistletoe (*Viscum album*) are evergreen, semi-parasitic shrubs which grow on various kinds of trees, mostly deciduous. The birds spread the seeds to other trees when eating its ripe red berries.

The Celts and Teutons held mistletoe in special esteem as a magic plant. To them it was invariably linked to the oak, their sacred tree. Celtic Druids used to gather it to use in their fertility rites because to them it symbolized regeneration and the restoration of family life.

American mistletoe is not recommended for medicinal purposes, while European mistletoe does not show any side effects when used as a medicine. European mistletoe acts on the circulatory system, first raising the blood pressure and then lowering it below the initial level. It is also used for arteriosclerosis and to stimulate the glandular activity related to digestion.

Cellular mistletoe juice contains all the inherent elements of the freshly gathered leafy twigs of the shrub in solution, not just one solitary element. These elements are: choline, a glycoside, an alkaloid, resin-like bitters, glucose and a substance with non-toxic action similar to digitalis, but much milder. These combined qualities produce the beneficial healing effect.

Man's well-being is based on several important prerequisites — primarily good circulation, closely linked to the nervous system. For these areas, fresh-pressed mistletoe juice is extremely effective.

As a therapy, mistletoe juice should be taken for several weeks in conjunction with a strictly vegetarian diet free of salt, alcohol, coffee, tea and tobacco. In order to increase the effects of mistletoe, the therapy should be complemented by a follow-up with hawthorn juice.

## **Oats**
### *The best restorative for nervous exhaustion*

Oats (*Avena sativa*) belong to the vast grain family – the original staple food of mankind. Oatmeal is still a favorite daily breakfast in Scotland and Canada and oats are part of Bircher-Muesli in Switzerland and the rest of Europe. It is decidedly a wholesome food with natural healing properties.

Grains are symbolically related in our minds to nature and its rhythmic cycles and forces. Ancient cultures lived according to these cycles, while twentieth century man, no longer attuned to nature, is often only conscious of the need to "go back to nature" when his "un-natural" mode of life has a disruptive effect on his health. In this connection, oats can be of real help for the restoration of soothing sleep and for calming frayed or exhausted nerves.

In Roman times, oats were mainly prescribed for diarrhea and as a general strengthening nutrient. Paracelsus praised oats as a splendid, nourishing food for the healthy and the ailing alike. It was only in medieval times that the wise herbalist, Mathiolas, first recommended oat-straw for external applications. It proved excellent for alleviating gout, rheumatism, skin rashes and liver complaints.

Today's oat juice is pressed from the fresh green plant at its most succulent stage – just before ripening. At this point in the plant's growth, certain qualities are retained in the juice, which would be lost at a later stage of development.

Oat juice merits attention as a natural sedative, capable of counteracting nervous irritability and lack of appetite. It is particularly recommended for convalescents after influenza and virus infections, in cases of nervous insomnia and as a tonic in states of exhaustion.

The ingredients have not yet been scientifically attested, but it is presently believed that oat juice contains several types of sugars (pentosane), vitamins and proteins, silica and other minerals as well as nitrogenous substances.

# Onion
## *A versatile home remedy through the millennia*

Mural paintings in pyramids lead one to the conclusion that the onion was sacred to the Egyptians. Similar to garlic, the onion probably originated in Central Asia. The Mediterranean countries used it as a staple food and the Romans spread it throughout their empire under the name *caepula*, which is the root of its present botanical name (*Allium cepa*). The medicinal part of the plant is the bulb.

When comparing folklore symbolism on a global basis, we learn that the motif of the "onion shape" is a symbol of growth and evolution in general. Old Egyptian pillars, East Indian and Chinese ornaments, Arabic frescoes, the steeples of Greek Orthodox churches and the world-famous Meissner porcelain from Germany all reveal the onion theme in many variations.

The onion contains a considerable amount of sulphuric etheric oils which stimulate the mucus membranes of the digestive organs. The result is an increased flow of digestive juices and greater absorption of nutrients. Onion juice prevents putrefactive and fermentation processes and inhibits the growth of harmful coliflora in the intestines. It is said to "thin" the blood – no doubt by purifying it – and to stimulate the bile flow.

Onion juice is used most often as a diuretic or expectorant agent, but it has also been used throughout the ages to relieve cramps, strengthen the heart, to expel worms and as a diuretic.

Mixed with honey, onion juice is good for hoarseness and coughs. Externally, it can be applied to infected wounds which will then heal in an astonishingly short time.

*He who has health has hope;*
*and he who has hope has everything.*

*Arabian proverb*

## Paprika, Red or Green Pepper
### *Rich in vitamin C*
### *and a tonic for heart and circulation*

Paprika (*Capsicum frutescens*) comes from the dried pods of the largest and mildest varieties of capsicum shrubs. (Its "hotter" relatives give us cayenne and chili powder.) Different varieties of paprika vary in quality and pungency. Some of the best originate from Hungary.

When buying paprika for juicing, ensure that they are grown organically. Most natural food stores offer California-grown paprika (peppers) year-round.

Paprika played a prominent part in the discovery of vitamins. Vitamin C was first isolated from it, as was vitamin P – which we now know as the bioflavonoids.

In natural paprika juice the vitamin C and bioflavonoid content is well balanced and valuable not only as nourishment, but also for its beneficial effects on the heart and circulation. The inherent balance of sodium and potassium also alleviates water retention.

In liquefied form, the paprika pod (pepper bell) is especially easy to assimilate for the debilitated or ailing patient.

# Parsley
## *More than a culinary herb*

Parsley (*Petroselinum sativum*) has its homeland in Greece and Sicily, and was used mainly as a medicinal plant throughout the middle ages. Its diuretic properties were highly valued, in addition to its ability to stimulate and strengthen the digestive organs and the whole glandular system, including the liver and spleen. Parsley juice also regulates the menstrual cycle.

"Sweet and beneficial to the stomach is parsley," wrote Galen in 1775, and today biochemists echo his views. It is interesting to note that only 50 years ago parsley was used by the medical profession – especially the French – as medicine.

Parsley leads the list of vegetables rich in iron. It is also rich in copper, manganese and vitamin $B_1$. As a low starch vegetable (7.4 percent), it helps to balance a concentrated starch or protein meal. Laboratory tests isolated etheric oils in the plant, root and seeds, of which *apiol* (parsley camphor) is the most important.

Because it is very potent, parsley juice should never be taken undiluted in large quantities. Dilute it in a proportion of one tablespoon to five or six tablespoons of liquid. Perhaps even blend it with carrot, celery or lettuce juice.

**Caution:** Parsley juice is not to be used *at all* if kidney inflammation exists, nor during pregnancy.

# Plantain or Ribwort
## *Helps clear up mucus congestion*

This well-known "weed," familiar to us all, grows in meadows and along roadsides. Plantain or ribwort (*Plantago lanceolata*) was used as a medicinal plant over 2,000 years ago to prevent bleeding, for blood cleansing, cramps, fever, gastritis, enteritis and as an expectorant. One of its more prominent proponents was Paracelsus who praised the plant's drying and astringent effect on tissues.

A chemical analysis shows the presence of trace elements, enzymes and a glycoside – *aucubin* – which merits special attention as an antibiotic. The latter is fully preserved in the stabilized cellular ribwort juice. Plantain, like the dandelion, assimilates traces of zinc from the soil. It also contains organic acids, saccharides and tannins. Probably the combination of these various substances in their natural proportion accounts for plantain juice's therapeutic effect. An analysis of minerals found in the ashes of this plant reveals the presence of potassium, sodium, calcium, magnesium, iron, phosphorus, sulphur and silicones, with a marked preponderance of potassium and silica.

Modern application of plantain juice is essentially based on its outstanding anti-inflammatory qualities in acute as well as chronic mucus congestion of the respiratory tract. It also yields excellent results with persistent catarrhs of the bronchial tube.

As part of the spring cleansing and blood rejuvenating juice therapy, plantain juice is successfully combined with nettle, dandelion and celery juice. Together they effect a general purification and energizing of the whole system.

*See: Respiratory Tract Therapy*

*Our life is frittered away by detail. . . . Simplify, simplify.*

*Henry David Thoreau*

# Potato
## *A benefactor to your stomach*

This "nightshade" plant hails from America and took a long time before it was whole-heartedly accepted as a staple food in Europe. Nowadays the potato (*Solanum tuberosum*) is part of most meals, particularly since modern nutritional research has discovered its value: 22 percent of its weight is easily digestible starch. A complex carbohydrate, its relatively high mineral content is comprised of potassium, calcium, magnesium and phosphorus. In addition the potato is very rich in vitamin C and high in fibre.

We know today that potato in the form of fresh-pressed juice has a healing effect on an overly acidic stomach. Potato juice is highly recommended in conjunction with other juices, including nettle and artichoke, for an overall body cleanse. However, it is important to prepare and take the juice shortly before the meal. Potato juice is a mild laxative and should be taken regularly for 10 to 14 days. The complaints of an acidic digestive tract will then quickly disappear. You will notice losing some weight, especially with a primarily vegetarian diet during the cleansing days.

It goes without saying, that all detrimental influences (such as alcohol, nicotine, as well as psychological conflicts, tension, stress, and worry) are to be avoided in order to effect a quick and positive reaction.

Potato juice can be diluted with cumin or camomile tea, thus improving the taste. Specific healing agents are the mucus ingredients as soluble fibre, vitamin C as an anti-inflammatory and antioxidant and some *solanin*-type ingredients which are concentrated under the potato skin. Freshly pressed juice from organically grown potatoes can be found in health food stores.

*See: Slimming/Weight Reducing Therapy*

# Pumpkin
## *The silent healer*

The field pumpkin or gourd (*Cucurbita pepo*) is a native of Mexico and was brought to Europe via Spain about 500 years ago. It is most popular in the southern regions around the Mediterranean Sea.

Pumpkin juice is of great importance in the renal (kidney) diet because of its elimination effect. All types of pumpkins act as mild laxatives and diuretics and remove dangerous intestinal toxins. Anyone who needs to take care of his/her urinary tract will do well to use cellulose-free, fresh-pressed pumpkin juice.

In order not to overtax the renal and urinary canals, a supplementation of natural vitamin C, such as acerola juice, should be added, observing an appropriate diet low in salt.

Just as in the case of the artichoke, pumpkin juice justifies the statement of Hippocrates: "Let your food be your medicine." Recently, intensive studies seemed to indicate that certain stimulating and anti-toxic elements might be in pumpkin juice. While isolation of these elements still eludes the chemists, they did find fats, sugars, proteins and a number of organic substances in pumpkin juice which aid the body's natural detoxification processes. Also, traces of vitamins and minerals, such as sodium, potassium, calcium, silica, magnesium, iron, sulphur and phosphorus, were identified.

Pumpkin juice is derived from the whole fresh pumpkin, including all the soluble ingredients of the pulp and the seeds.

*Unless we change direction,*
*we are likely to end up*
*where we are headed.*

*Chinese proverb*

# Ramson
## *A "wild" cousin of the garlic family*

This pretty plant is found in damp and shady woods, usually in lime-rich soil. It is known all over Europe by the name of "bear's garlic" *(Allium ursinum)*, and can be found under shade-providing hedges and in cool lofty forests, where it soon reveals itself by its pungent odor.

Dioscorides mentioned this plant as an effective blood purifier. It is still used in that capacity today. Ramson is not only equal to the cultivated garlic, but is in many ways superior because of its truly natural ingredients, unspoiled by the good intentions of man's cultivating hands.

Walther Schoenenberger succeeded in stabilizing fresh-pressed, cellular ramson juice and making it nearly odorless, without affecting in the least the efficacy of its etheric sulphuric oils, minerals and vitamins.

Cellular ramson juice is said to be helpful for general improvement of the circulatory system, for liver problems, and in arteriosclerosis (even in advanced stages). For getting rid of pinworms in children, dilute one tablespoonful of ramson juice with one quarter litre of water as an enema.

Ramson juice is particularly recommended for gastro-intestinal catarrh, diarrhea and constipation, as well as for emphysema with bronchitis. It has been found to effect a slow, long-lasting lowering of blood pressure. In general, it can be used like garlic juice.

Recommended particularly for gastro-intestinal complaints of bacterial origin, it is also good for *Candida albicans* (yeast infection). It is most effective when combined with wormwood juice. It is similarly recommended for high blood pressure due to arteriosclerosis.

*Wisdom is knowing what to do; virtue is doing it.*

*Chinese proverb*

# Red Beets
## *Their multiple effects are still to be explored*

The ancient Greeks and Romans used red beets (*Beta conditiva alef*) as a remedy for fever complaints. In medieval times, the juice of red beet roots was recommended as an easily digestible food during various illnesses.

It seems to have been an effective digestive regulator for centuries. The purifying and nourishing qualities of red beets have always been of great value to the nutritionist, and there is unanimous agreement among naturopaths about the fever-reducing, disinfecting, loosening and eliminating properties of this vegetable. Beets obviously stimulate and strengthen the peristaltic activity of the bowels as well as the neighboring glands: liver, gallbladder, spleen and kidneys.

The bright red color of the beet – which seems to indicate large stores of vitamins and minerals – attracted the attention of modern medical and nutritional researchers. Their laboratory tests authenticated the claims of our forebears. Thus, red beets are recommended today as an easily digestible food (containing carbohydrates, vitamins and minerals) for cases of weakness, sensitive stomach, and for stimulation of the kidneys.

Red beets particularly stimulate the function of the lymphatic system and strengthen bodily resistance to infection in young adults. Because of their general fever-reducing and nourishing effect, red beets have a most favorable influence on catarrhs in connection with colds and flu. Furthermore, red beets speed up the metabolism and facilitate digestion.

As a nutritional supplement in cases of cancer, red beets have gained a reputation in recent years, due to the research carried out by Drs. Ferenczi, Seeger and Trub. Their tests and results have been chronicled in many scientific publications, particularly in the book *Red Beets as Therapeutical Supplement for Patients with Malignant Growths* (Karl F. Haug Verlag, Heidelberg.)

The red beet juice made by Walther Schoenenberger, available in health food stores, is pressed from organically grown beets which contain large amounts of alkaline lime, potassium, phosphorus and easily digestible natural sugars, in addition to the red pigment. Worth mentioning also is the choline, which stimulates peristalsis of the intestines.

It should be said here that commercially available red beet powders are often produced for only one purpose: food coloring. Therefore, not much attention is paid to organic cultivation for the preservation of naturally occurring organic materials. Commercially grown beets should be avoided for therapeutic purposes.

Dr. Ferenczi's red beet diet calls for great quantities of beets or beet juice and, for this reason, the scientific department of the Schoenenberger plant juice company has developed a drying process which produces instant beet powder in which the natural pigment and all the organic substances are preserved. In this process, the beet juice is atomized into a vacuum, the liquid evaporated and the dry, heavier residue then collected. Only organically grown red beets are used to produce these red beet powder crystals which are easily diluted with water to reconstitute the juice.

# Rosehips
## *Five times more vitamin C than lemon*

The wild rose (*Rosa canina*) grows in several varieties all over Europe and North and Central America, providing us with fruit each autumn – shiny red rosehips. The sprawling bushes with the pretty pink rose-like blooms are to be found at the edges of forests, ravines, roadsides or along fences.

In past centuries, rosehips were used as tea infusions for various ailments which are today classified as avitaminosis (vitamin deficiency). Present-day research has shown that this fruit, so exceedingly rich in vitamin C (five times as much as the lemon), should only be used fresh since 90 percent of this precious vitamin is lost when the rosehips are dried. This natural source of vitamin C has proven far superior to a synthetic supplement, mainly due to the other vitamins contained in the fruit. Rosehips are, therefore, an ideal natural multi-vitamin, containing beta-carotene (precursor of vitamin A), vitamins $B_1$, $B_2$, C, K, E, bioflavonoids, fructose, fruit acids and special aromatic substances.

At first, vitamin C was prescribed for symptoms of scurvy and related bleeding gums and loosening of teeth. But nowadays nutritionists see a much greater value in vitamin C. A lack of this vitamin, for instance, is partly to blame for our "spring fatigue," which is a weak immune system manifested in lowered resistance to colds, chills and infections.

In some parts of North America, rosehips grow abundantly and can be collected in a very short time. To remove the kernels will take some time though, but the resulting juice or jam is most beneficial.

The somewhat acidic flavor of the rosehip juice can be improved by the addition of apricot juice, which at the same time raises the vitamin A content. So regardless of the season, whenever a "spring fatigue" overcomes you, it is recommended that you take a small glass of undiluted rosehip-apricot juice three to four times daily. This juice, by the way, gives you the additional benefits of being both a mild laxative and a mild diuretic.

# Rosemary
## *A natural stimulant for nerves and circulation*

This evergreen shrub, originating in the Mediterranean area, is now widely cultivated for both its aromatic leaves and its use as a seasoning. Since rosemary (*Rosmarinus officinalis*) is sensitive to frost and does not grow wild in northern latitudes, special measures must be taken for its successful cultivation.

Rosemary offers something special in our native plant world. Part of its fragrance comes from the camphor – in no way secondary to the Japanese camphor tree – and it is mainly this ingredient which stimulates the heart and circulation. The old herbal books put it this way: "Rosemary makes you bold and lively." The juice of this herb belongs in the class of restoratives and natural stimulants. It also acts favorably on the functions of the liver, the production of bile, and proper digestion in general.

Pure rosemary juice is recommended particularly for the elderly who have weak circulation. Additional external stimulation to the circulation can be achieved by dry-brushing the whole body with a loofah, as well as alternating hot and cold showers or baths.

# Sage
## *A "saviour and healing mediator of nature"*

Sage (*Salvia officinalis*) is indigenous to the South, where it grows wild in great profusion. In our northern regions, garden sage has been mainly cultivated since the first medieval monastery gardens.

Ancient botanists were keenly aware of this plant's many healing qualities, as witnessed by the Latin name *salvia*, stemming from *salvare*, meaning "to heal." The Hippocratic physicians, Dioscorides and Galen, used sage to build blood and for its diuretic, menstruation-regulating and general tonic properties. Walefrid Strabo apparently popularized this plant in the fourteenth century, so that it found its way into farmers' gardens and was widely used in folk medicine. Paracelsus reinforced its fame with his own experiments, and ever since then sage has been among the best known medicinal plants. The reputation of this plant is best expressed in the praise bestowed upon it by the medical school in Salerno, Italy: *"Salvia salvatrix, naturae conciliatrix,"* meaning "Sage, you saviour and healing mediator of nature."

Sage juice is derived from the flowering plant at its highest peak of etheric oil content. This oil gives the plant its typical scent.

Sage's best known effect is the suppression of perspiration, which usually begins about two hours after taking sage juice, tea or tincture, and may last for several days. This property makes it useful for night sweats, such as those common with tuberculosis. A nursing mother whose child has just been weaned can take sage tea or juice for a few days to help stop the flow of milk.

Cellular sage juice is indicated for nervous conditions, exhaustion, trembling, depression and vertigo. As an astringent, it can be used for diarrhea, gastritis and enteritis. As a gargle, in diluted form, it is good for healing a sore throat, laryngitis and tonsillitis. It also helps to eliminate mucus congestion in the respiratory passages and the stomach.

## Sauerkraut
### *The best friend your digestive system could wish for*

Father Kneipp called sauerkraut "the best friend of your digestive organs." He also declared in his famous work *Thus Should You Live,*[1] published in 1886: "those who regularly partake of sauerkraut will live longest!" This tells us that sauerkraut has a most beneficial effect on our health, staving off old age. But how is this possible?

To make sauerkraut, green cabbage (*Brassica oleracea var. capita*) is finely shredded, salted with sea salt and seasoned with mustard seed and juniper berries before it is allowed to undergo a natural lactic acid fermentation in clean wooden barrels or special fermentation crocks. The lactic acid in sauerkraut is approximately 20 percent (D-) and 80 percent (L+). It is precisely this (L+) lactic acid that so beneficially affects the general digestion, by disinfecting the stomach and colon as well as inhibiting the growth of certain harmful bacteria which cause putrefaction, flatulence and even toxicity. In addition, analyses testify that sauerkraut has a considerable content of mineral salts and trace elements, such as potassium, calcium, phosphorus, iron, copper, plus vitamin C. Sauerkraut, like natural, unsweetened yogurt, also provides (L+) lactic bacteria, the friendly flora for human intestines.

---

[1] *So sollt Ihr leben.*

Let us not forget, then, that a copious intake of sauerkraut or sauerkraut juice is most beneficial for our digestion, blood regeneration and the metabolism of the whole system. A daily glass of sauerkraut juice ought to be considered an excellent preventative measure against cancer, gout, rheumatism and premature aging. Dr. Johannes Kuhl, a famous German cancer researcher, maintains that the lack of (L+) lactic acid in our modern diet is the cause of the widespread incidence of cancer.

For further reading I highly recommend *Making sauerkraut and pickled vegetables at home* by Annelies Schoeneck, published by alive books.

*If the Germans ate as much*
*sauerkraut as the French*
*believe they do, they would*
*have no cancer.*

*Johannes Kuhl, MD*

# Silverweed
## *An anti-spasmodic juice*

Among the Greek physicians of antiquity, it was Theophrastus who highly praised the silverweed *(Potentilla anserina)* and old herbal books have carried its fame as the popularly known "cramp weed" since then. This, incidentally, describes the fresh plant's most common medicinal use.

Historically, herbalists recommended silverweed for dropsy, jaundice, liver and spleen ailments, and for menstrual difficulties. Furthermore, it seems to have a favorable effect on various stomach complaints and cramp-causing intestinal ailments, such as colic and diarrhea. It is also good for dysentery.

Silverweed juice is rich in minerals and contains a natural anti-spasmodic ingredient, thus making it the obvious natural remedy for cramp relief, a replacement for the poisonous, yet frequently used, drug, atropin. Silverweed juice is frequently combined with camomile juice or peppermint tea. It is also useful as an external astringent for skin problems, mouth and throat sores, and similar complaints.

# Spinach
## *Builds blood and restores cells*

Spinach (*Spinacea oleracea*) is esteemed as much for its tastiness as for its nutritional and medicinal value. Like that of the carrot, spinach juice is tolerated even by babies of six months.

Spinach is native to northern Africa, brought to Europe via Spain by the Arabs. As with all other green-leaf vegetables, spinach supplies us with chlorophyll, which has a great affinity with the hemoglobin in our blood. The rich content of vitamins A, B, C and E, and minerals (headed by iron, but also including potassium, calcium, sodium, magnesium, phosphorus, sulphates and traces of iodine, nickel and cobalt) place spinach as the number one vegetable for deficiency diseases. It is exceptionally rich in the blood-building factor folic acid (part of the vitamin B complex) which is further supported by its high content of easily assimilated iron. Because of these ingredients, spinach juice is recommended in cases of anemia, general weakness, convalescence, rheumatism and arthritis.

Spinach juice has a favorable influence on general digestion, especially on the action of the intestines. It is equally highly recommended for strengthening the nervous system, useful as a tonic for those doing intensive mental work and for people who complain about cold hands and feet.

# St. John's Wort
## *Strengthens your nerves*

The old Latin name for St. John's Wort is *Hypericum perforatum*, which is derived from the Greek and the Roman physicians who were among those using this plant for natural therapies. Dioscorides, Hippocrates and Plinius are just three of the most outstanding names of that period.

Among the physicians of the Middle Ages who treated patients with this nerve-soothing and strengthening plant is Paracelsus. He held it in highest esteem as an ointment for sores or wounds when mixed with honey. In the nineteenth century, St. John's Wort was still being used in this form as well as for cases of manic depression. Homeopaths have never ceased to rely on this plant for its calming and restorative powers.

At present, because of the research of Walther Schoenenberger, St. John's Wort's value is emphasized more and more as a specific nerve tonic for cases of depression and nervous exhaustion caused by overstrain. The juice is particularly effective as a nervine, whereas the dried herbs have lost the specific active ingredient of the red pigment, *hypericin*, reducing their soothing and strengthening effect on the nerves. It has been said that this pigment literally "feeds" the energy of the sun to the nerves and glands. The superiority of cellular juice versus dried herbs can be especially demonstrated with St. John's Wort.

Cellular St. John's Wort juice is also a beneficial curative in cases of neuralgia, headache and rheumatism if not caused by severe organic deficiencies. Nervous restlessness, insomnia and overactivity of the thyroid are favorably influenced by St. John's Wort juice, particularly when taken in conjunction with valerian juice and lycopus juice as a therapeutic approach. Nervousness, cramps and menstrual difficulties call for the natural healing therapy of St. John's Wort juice, supported by valerian juice.

*See: Nerve Restorative Therapy*

## Stinging Nettle
### *Stimulates your metabolism*

Stinging nettles are plants which grow only near human habitation and flourish in areas where scrap iron has been discarded – such as behind barns and in dumps. Apparently a weed, the nettle family (*Urtica dioica*) nevertheless sets high demands on the soil, requiring considerable amounts of nitrogen and specific mineral content. The nettle enjoyed an enviable reputation in ancient times. Dioscorides ascribed diuretic qualities to it, as did the Roman herbalists Plinius, Amatus and Sartorius. The healing fame of nettles was upheld throughout the Middle Ages.

Having passed the critical analyses of the twentieth century pharmaceutical sciences with great honors, the nettle's stimulating effects on the kidneys and its resulting diuretic effects are medically proven. The external use of the fresh stinging nettle leaves in cases of rheumatism is well known even today. The stinging feeling on the skin surface left by the etheric oils of the leaves is equal to an injection of formic acid.

However, one of the best known and acclaimed uses of natural, fresh-pressed nettle juice is as a blood purifier. Walther Schoenenberger's experiments and tests have shown that nettle juice stimulates the metabolism, thereby dissolving waste products in the system and – because of its diuretic properties – flushing them out. Since both dissolving and flushing actions are most important for the purification of

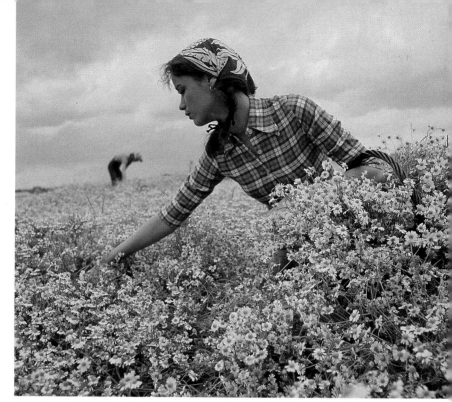

▲ Harvesting Camomile

▼ Flowering Borage

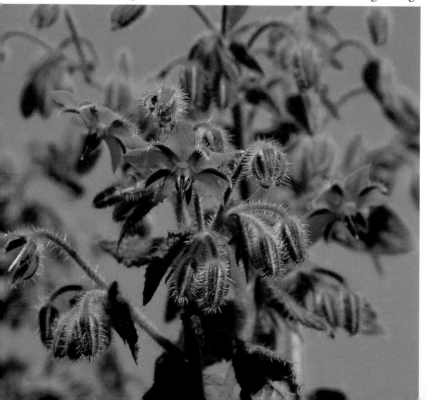

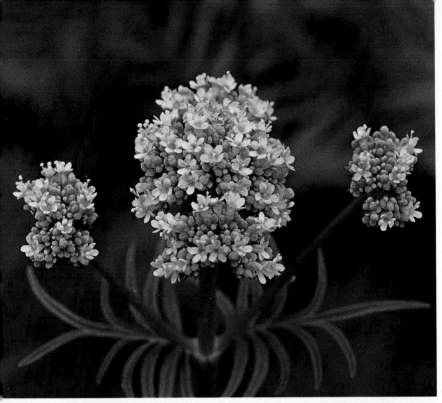

▲ Valerian Blossoms

▼ St. John's Wort

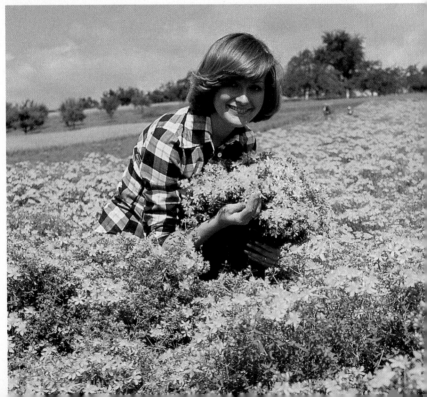

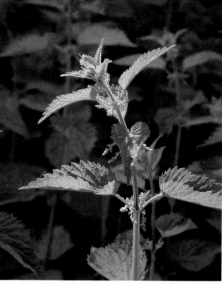

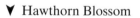
▲ Stinging Nettle

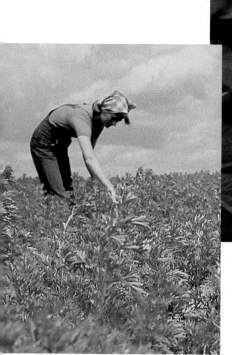

▲ Wormwood                    ▼ Hawthorn Blossom

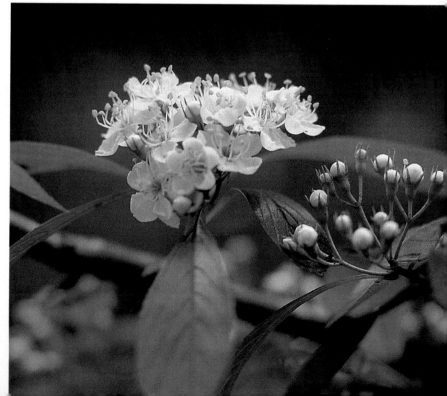

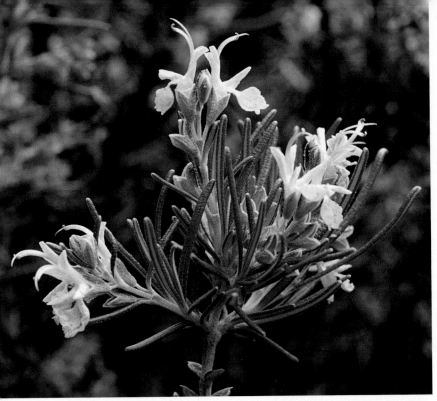

▲ Rosemary in Bloom   ▼ A Field of Garden Sage

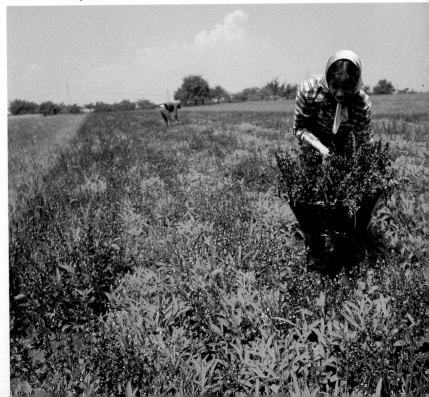

the blood, stinging nettle juice is the remedy *par excellence* for all complaints where toxicity and/or over-acidity of the blood are part of the problem source, including rheumatism and arthritis. Given its propensity to dissolve and flush waste, nettle juice is also a "natural" for weight reduction.

But let us not forget the tonic and restorative properties of this wondrous medicinal "weed." Because of the nettle's high mineral content and blood building properties, it is particularly recommended for degenerative diseases and old age symptoms. Nettle juice is similarly recommended in cases of anemia. Because of its high iron content, nettle juice rivals the effectiveness of spinach juice.

These blood-restorative qualities are only inherent in fresh-pressed nettle juice. They are NOT present in the dried herb used for infusions because the medicinal oils evaporate in the drying process. In fact, stinging nettle best illustrates the change in composition of ingredients which every herb undergoes during the drying process. While it is almost impossible to handle the fresh plant without gloves because of its burning effects, within fifteen minutes after the plant is cut down you can touch it without any stinging sensation; the etheric oils have already evaporated. For this reason, the juice, which captures this medicinal ingredient, is more effective than the dried herb.

Nursing mothers can also assure a sufficient quantity of milk by using fresh-pressed cellular nettle juice. Due to the stimulation of gland secretions, particularly those of the digestive tract, various eczemas can be cleared up by the use of this juice. Nettle juice also alleviates the discomforts of hemorrhoids and facilitates bowel evacuation.

Chemical tests of nettle juice have shown that, in addition to various interesting organic substances (sugars, histamine-like ingredients, vitamins and secretines), it has a very high mineral content. When burned, the residue contains lime, potassium, iron, manganese, titanium, chlorine, phosphorus and sulphur.

*See: Blood Purifying Therapy; Regenerative Therapy;*
*   Slimming/Weight Reducing Therapy*

*Whatsoever a man soweth;*
*so shall he reap.*

*Galatians 6:7*

# Thyme
## *A soothing anti-spasmodic*

Though hailing from Mediterranean shores, thyme (*Thymus vulgaris*) has been known throughout Europe, even up to the far North, since the eleventh century. Both ancient and contemporary herbalists speak lovingly of this small, shrubby plant, with its strong, spicy taste and odor. No wonder that thyme was extensively cultivated throughout the centuries and found in most kitchen gardens – ready for quick treatment of throat and bronchial problems, chronic gastritis, laryngitis or whooping cough. The oldest herbal prescriptions specify "for coughs and spasmodic complaints, make the medication from the *fresh* plant." A warm infusion was said to promote perspiration and relieve flatulence and colic.

Because of its powerful antiseptic action, oil of thyme (*thymol*) is used in mouthwashes and toothpastes. Thyme baths are said to be helpful for rheumatic problems, neurasthenia, paralysis, bruises, swelling and sprains. A salve made from thyme has been used for shingles.

Fresh-pressed cellular thyme juice is beneficial for all respiratory complaints. *Thymol* not only helps to clean mucus congestion from the lungs and respiratory passages, but simultaneously disinfects them as well. Thyme juice also makes a good tonic for the stomach and nerves, and is used for gastro-intestinal problems, such as mild gastritis, enteritis, stomach cramps and painful menstruation.

For the strengthening of respiratory passages, a therapeutic combination of thyme juice, plantain juice and coltsfoot juice is highly efficacious.

*To the man who is truly ethical
all life is sacred, including that which,
from the human point of view,
seems lower in the scale.*

*Albert Schweitzer*

# Tomato
## *A harmonious set of vitamins*

The nightshade family of plants spread from the Americas to the rest of the world mainly through three of its representatives: the potato, tobacco and the tomato. Ever since its rich vitamin content was discovered, the tomato has been mass-cultivated and placed on the "must" list of all health-conscious people.

The tomato (*Lycopersicon esculentum*) is native to Peru. Its name is apparently of Mexican origin and means "apple of paradise" or "apple of life." The Portuguese were probably the first to bring the plant to the Mediterranean regions. From there it spread to Turkey and the Orient, as well as across the Balkans to the rest of Europe where it soon became a popular food and spice.

The therapeutic and nutrient value of the tomato lies primarily in its high vitamin content, particularly vitamins A and C. Its vitamin B content is also considerable. Tomatoes also contain traces of vitamin D and the bioflavonoids. Organically grown field tomatoes are the most desirable – whole, as pulp or in juice form. In addition to organic acids, the tomato also has an astounding mixture of minerals, such as calcium, phosphorus, potassium, manganese, and traces of iron, copper and cobalt.

This combination of vitamins and minerals, plus *saponin* and some oxalic acid, favorably stimulates the digestive juices, particularly the pancreas. The tomato is mildly laxative, soothes cramps (because of its magnesium content), is well tolerated by the ailing liver – and has very few calories! Therefore, it is often recommended for a juice fasting cleanse to supply all essential vitamins without adding calories.

Tomato juice should be given to children who are anemic due to iron deficiency. When combined with spinach juice and carrot juice, the effects of enriched blood will soon be noted in the form of rosy cheeks, for example. Tomato juice is further recommended to improve appetite, for expectant and nursing mothers, for convalescents, and for cases of general weakness due to vitamin deficiency.

Tomato juice for therapeutic use must not be salted as sodium promotes water retention within the cells.

*See: Slimming/Weight Reducing Therapy*

# Valerian
## *Soothing for the nerves*

This plant can look back on a centuries-old history as a medicinal herb. Valerian (*Valeriana officinalis*) was known by the Greeks, used extensively in medieval herb lore, and was highly valued by the physicians of the fifteenth and sixteenth centuries. Its use as a healing, soothing herb for nervous conditions, and as a diuretic and perspirant, continued throughout the ages to the twentieth century.

The soothing effect stems from the plant's various etheric oils and also from some of the ingredients in the roots. In cases of insomnia, nervous exhaustion and excessive mental stress, the multiple sedative reactions of valerian juice on the nervous system and the digestive tract make it a most valuable natural remedy with no side effects or dangers of addiction. It effectively replaces chemical or synthetic sleeping pills and tranquilizers. In cases of a tendency toward spasms, such as in menstrual disturbances, nervous spasms of the gastro-intestinal tract or nerve-related headaches, this juice is very calming.

The pure cellular juice, pressed from the fresh rhizomes of the valerian plant, and available at your health food store, contains no chemicals or added water. It is almost scentless and tasteless. Valerian juice is a perfect, manifold, natural sedative which finds an excellent complement in the nerve-restorative qualities of St. John's Wort juice.

*See: Nerve Restorative Therapy*

# Watercress
## *The ideal spring tonic*

Not only did the ancient Greeks and Romans cherish watercress (*Nasturtium officinalis*) but, according to the famous Greek writer Xenophon, the Persians used to eat quantities of it raw when subjected to heavy physical labor. Medieval herbalists were well aware of its blood cleansing and restorative properties, not to mention its stimulating effect on the spleen, liver and gallbladder. Since ancient times, watercress has been part of spring cleansing therapies, the chief aim of which is to purify the blood and rejuvenate winter-sluggish bodies by expelling toxins from the body. Many skin irritations and eczemas, which originate in metabolic impurities, disappear upon treatment with watercress juice. Lately, the stimulating effect of this juice on kidney metabolism has been particularly emphasized.

Watercress has an exceptionally high mineral content, paralleled by high alkalinity. Its possible effect on the glandular system is due to sulphuric oils and iodine content and the mustard-like, pungent oils that increase the elimination of waste products. The high vitamin C content is most surprising, but this could be considered an additional deciding factor for choosing watercress juice as an ideal spring tonic, since we have a great need of vitamin C at this time of year.

Watercress is best used raw as part of a salad and, of course, as fresh-pressed juice. The latter is available throughout the year in health food stores.

When combined with nettle juice, the properties of watercress juice are reinforced, providing an effective blood cleansing, restorative and energizing spring tonic.

*See: Slimming/Weight Reducing Therapy*

*Come forth into*
*the light of things,*
*Let nature be your teacher.*

*William Wordsworth*

# Wormwood
## *A tried and true friend for over 4,000 years*

The Greeks knew it as a classic medicine, and the Romans prescribed it. And Paracelsus (to mention one medieval celebrity) testified to its efficacy. The seventeenth century physicians of France used it as a stomach remedy in cases of appetite loss, debilitation of gastro-intestinal functions, and as a stimulant of the liver and gallbladder. Wormwood (*Artemisia absinthium*) stimulates gallbladder secretions because of the bitter compound contained in its etheric oils.

Every so often, wormwood comes under attack from government bodies because of its apparent content of *thujon*, a substance said to cause hallucinations. You may rest assured that *thujon* presents absolutely no problem with fresh pressed cellular juices or with herbal teas. *Thujon* is alcohol-soluble only and needs to be taken in enormously large quantities to cause any adverse reaction.

The benefits of wormwood stem from its high concentration of bitters. Empirical evidence has established wormwood as a valuable medicinal herb that has been used for centuries.

It has also long been established that the taste of fresh wormwood juice is much superior to that of tea. The juice generally promotes gastric function, especially in cases of hyper- and hypo-acidity, heartburn, lack of appetite, stomach upsets, flatulence and gastric-intestinal mucus inflammation.

Bad breath, headache, dysentery and formation of gas will also be beneficially influenced.

Wormwood juice combined with silverweed juice acts favorably on inflammatory-catarrhal complaints of the gastrointestinal tract. In cases of colic or lazy colon, alternate wormwood juice with dandelion and black radish juice.

*See: Stomach and Intestinal Problems Therapy*

## Yarrow
### *Improves the elasticity of blood vessels, strengthens muscles*

Yarrow (*Achillea millefolicium*) is a perennial plant found in waste places all over the world: fields, pastures, meadows and along railroad embankments or roadsides.

Yarrow tea has a long history of empirical evidence for treatment of appetite loss, stomach cramps, flatulence, gastritis, enteritis, gallbladder and liver problems and internal hemorrhage, particularly in the lungs.

Fresh yarrow juice acts as a general tonic and as a prophylactic (preventive treatment) by building blood. At the same time, it improves the elasticity of blood vessels and so facilitates not only the flow of blood to the surface of the skin, but also lets the heart work more efficiently while soothing the nerves.

Because of its particularly bitter properties, yarrow juice has a distinctive influence on tissues and muscles, especially in the lower back and pelvis regions where the female organs are situated. Because of this special therapy for women, yarrow is known as the "women's herb." It strengthens the veins, relieves mood changes during menopause, and relieves stomach and intestinal trouble.

An inclination toward irritability can often be overcome with a "tuning-up" therapy over a period of time, utilizing yarrow juice in conjunction with dandelion juice and borage or rosemary juice.

*See: Female Complaints Therapy; Stomach and Intestinal Problems Therapy*

*Good health is often
a matter of good judgement.*

*Marion D. Hanks*

*Honor the healer for his services,*
*For the Lord created him.*
*His skill comes from the Most High,*
*And he is rewarded by kings.*
*The healer's knowledge gives him standing*
*and wins him the admiration of the great.*
*The Lord has created medicines from the earth,*
*And a sensible man will not disparage them.*

*Apocrypha, Ecclesiasticus 38:1–4*

# IV

# Herbal Juice Therapies
# for Specific Ailments

*Fresh-pressed juices assist the weakened physical body.
Ever so subtly, they counteract the slow process
of deterioration, purify the constantly
overburdened organism, strengthen it, and thereby
help build up resistance to serious diseases.*

**Note:** In the following section of the book a combination of several different juices are recommended for the treatment of specific ailments. These treatment packages, designed for a duration of several days, are simply referred to as "therapy units." The juices and herbal teas recommended as a therapy unit should be consumed within the time period allocated, without interruption. One therapy unit may consist of three different juices. In cases where you start with one type of juice for the first three days and continue with another juice for the second three days, finish the first bottle of juice entirely before changing to another juice.

## Arteriosclerosis Therapy

How does arteriosclerosis come about? As long as arteries function as tubes transporting blood, they can be said to be adequate. However, in many people they are rendered inadequate by obstruction. A blockage within an artery often develops from fatty material (such as cholesterol) deposited along the lining of the artery to fill the crevices that have occurred due to "fraying" or degeneration. In the attempt to repair and strengthen the weakened walls, nature begins to deposit calcium. The long-term consequences, which increase with age, are a loss of elasticity and resilience of the arterial network, usually in some specific areas of the body, such as the heart, brain, kidneys and major blood vessels to the extremities. Thus, insufficient blood supplies reach the affected areas, eventually causing disease symptoms.

To relieve the aggravating symptoms of hardening of the arteries (arteriosclerosis) and to reduce cholesterol content and strengthen the heart, the following fresh-pressed cellular plant juices should be combined as an effective therapy over a period of three to four weeks:

> 2 bottles hawthorn juice
> 1 bottle garlic juice
> 1 package camomile herb tea

**Every day:**
Before breakfast:     1 tablespoon of hawthorn juice
                      with one cup of camomile tea

| Before lunch: | 1 tablespoon of hawthorn juice with $1/2$ cup of water |
|---|---|
| Before bedtime: | 1 tablespoon of hawthorn juice with one cup of water |
| **For first ten days** | also take 1 tablespoon of garlic juice with water or soup each day |

## The Prescribed Juices

Hawthorn juice is the most complementary remedy to garlic juice in this therapy. Its restorative and strengthening properties assist the function of the heart in all its aspects, and widen the blood vessels (dilatation) to allow for increased oxygen intake and a normalization of blood pressure.

Garlic juice acts favorably on the various symptoms of arteriosclerosis, such as dizziness, feelings of depression and anxiety, disturbed sleep and lack of concentration. The sulphuric etheric oil content in the garlic juice effects a change in the bacterial flora of the colon, minimizing putrefaction and increasing elimination of all toxic waste.

The above specified amounts and the type of juices or tea are considered a "therapy-unit." It is suggested to follow this up with one or two more units for greater effectiveness. In this manner, total energy will be extended over three to four weeks.

## Juice Fasting

For all those who are able to take time off for a complete rest, it is strongly recommended they schedule at least one day of juice fasting, either during the therapy or between therapy-units. This will greatly support and strengthen the effects of the plant juices, reduce stress on the heart and promote a feeling of general well-being.

On days of juice fasting nothing is taken except one litre (approximately one quart) of vegetable or fruit juices, including the prescribed therapeutic juices and tea. A very appropriate "fasting drink" is the vegetable weight-reducing "Lightning Cleanse" described on page 170, or you may prepare your own juice cocktail from fresh vegetables or fruits.[1]

## Diet

A very essential part of this therapy – or any therapy – is an appropriate diet rich in minerals, proteins, fresh raw vegetables and fruit, low in salt intake, with all saturated fats – including margarine – replaced by unrefined, cold-pressed, unsaturated oils.[2] Lecithin and soy beans will effectively minimize the cholesterol content of the blood, while the high fibre content of fresh whole foods contributes to the healthy activity of the eliminative system. Total abstinence from stimulants, particularly tobacco, is also required.

Flax oil is especially recommended as it is rich in both essential fatty acids, Omega 3, Omega 6, linoleic and linolenic fatty acids. The western civilized diet is deficient in both of these essential fatty acids and the absence of Omega 6 has been linked with both heart and circulatory problems.

---

[1] There are many good books published on juice fasting, highly recommended is *The Joy of Juice Fasting* by Klaus Kaufmann, published by *alive* books, Vancouver, BC, 1990.

[2] Depending on the country you live in, these natural unprocessed oils may be either easily obtained or hard to find. In any case, check with your local health food store. Further reading: *Fats that Heal – Fats that Kill* by Udo Erasmus, *alive* books, Vancouver, BC, 4th printing, 1991.

## Arthritis and Rheumatism Therapy

This therapy unit of plant juices is designed to neutralize the over-acidity of the system, to flush out retained excess fluids and all waste from the tissues, and to "tune-up" the whole organism. It is supposed to restore the proper acid/alkaline balance of the blood and soothe inflamed tissues. As a preventative measure, this therapy is recommended to all those who have a predisposition to arthritic-rheumatic complaints. For grave rheumatic illnesses, particularly when accompanied by fever, a nutrition-oriented physician should be consulted.

Arthritis and rheumatism are systemic diseases in which the whole organism is involved. The cause of the pain is usually found in poor blood circulation which results in an inadequate supply of blood sugar, oxygen, vitamins and salts to the tissues affected. Lack of exercise further aggravates this situation.

The way of natural therapy is to co-operate with your own body. Health is not a gift, but must be acquired, or recaptured, and then maintained. On this basis, the arthritis-rheumatism therapy endeavors to achieve three goals:

1. Increase elimination of the body wastes through birch juice and horseradish distillate.
2. Provide adequate nourishment, sufficient raw food and salt intake.
3. Start a more physically active lifestyle by doing moderate exercises.

The therapy unit consists of:

4 bottles of birch juice
2 bottles of horseradish distillate
2 packages of couch grass tea

**1st - 4th day**

Before breakfast:    1 cup couch grass tea with
1 tablespoon birch juice

Before lunch:    1 tablespoon horseradish distillate in
$1/2$ cup water

Before bedtime:    1 cup couch grass tea with
1 tablespoon horseradish distillate

**5th - 8th day**

Before breakfast:    1 cup couch grass tea with
1 tablespoon birch juice

Before lunch:    1 tablespoon birch juice in
$1/2$ cup water

Before bedtime:    1 cup couch grass tea with
1 tablespoon birch juice

**9th - 12th day**

Before breakfast:    1 cup couch grass tea with
1 tablespoon horseradish distillate

Before lunch:    1 tablespoon horseradish distillate
in $1/2$ cup water

Before bedtime:    1 cup couch grass tea with
1 tablespoon horseradish distillate

**13th – 24th day**

| | |
|---|---|
| Before breakfast: | 1 cup couch grass tea with 1 tablespoon birch juice |
| Before lunch: | 1 tablespoon birch juice in $1/2$ cup water |
| Before bedtime: | 1 cup couch grass tea with 1 tablespoon birch juice |

## The Prescribed Juices

Horseradish distillate stimulates the whole body metabolism due to its specific etheric oils, which are strongly diuretic. This latter effect is very helpful, since the benefits of arthritic-rheumatic treatments result mainly from the increased elimination of all wastes and toxins from the system.

Birch juice, thanks to its content of *saponins*, resins and etheric oils, also excels as a diuretic without irritating the kidneys. The results are purification of the blood as well as a flushing out of the distended and inflamed tissues.

Couch grass tea has, for centuries, been recommended by herbalists for arthritic-rheumatic complaints. Lately, due to the experiments of Walther Schoenenberger, it has been combined with the above-mentioned juices for greater effectiveness.

## Diet

A vital part of this therapy is the right kind of nourishment – such as an increase in alkaline-reactive foods, rich in vitamins and minerals. Vegetables, fruit, milk and salads are all high on the list of desirable foods, and most of them should be consumed raw. Black tea, coffee, chocolate and alcohol are, to the arthritic or rheumatic patient, dangerous stimulant poisons and should be avoided altogether.

It is further recommended to eliminate – at least for the duration of the therapy – all animal proteins (meat, fish, eggs), all dry legumes (beans, peas, lentils) and salt. In order to maintain improved health after termination of the therapy units (repeated two to three times and supplemented by a day of juice fasting), a reduced intake of all uric acid-forming foods (such as red meat and beef) should be the rule.

To eliminate uric acid from the body, Devil's Claw 410 Extract tablets from Dr. Dünner of Switzerland are recommended with the therapy unit of herbal juices. This herbal supplement, containing *harpagophite*, aids the stimulation of liver and gallbladder functions by ridding the body of uric acid which, when concentrated and crystallized within the joints, causes inflammation and painful swelling. Devil's Claw 410 Extract tablets are totally safe and without any known side effects.[1]

---

[1] Canada Health & Welfare Health Protection Branch, *Studies on Devil's Claw.*

## Blood Purification Therapy

No transportation system, either in nature or technology, deserves more admiration than the blood and the circulatory system of our bodies. It is the "traffic network" through which all ingredients, both consumed and absorbed, have to pass. With its many minor and major "supply avenues," the total length of one human circulatory system is more than double that of the earth's circumference!

However, the blood is not only the transportation system of our bodies, it is also a vigilant observer of our health. It can instantly repair minor mishaps, such as a cut in the finger, and the white blood corpuscles – the real "blood specialists" – neutralize or even expel such alien intruders as bacteria or poisons.

Since a sufficient blood supply provides the necessary nourishment and oxygen essential for the healthy upkeep and proper functioning of all organs, everything possible should be undertaken to maintain a proper blood flow, free from pollutants and other harmful substances. Fortunately, nature has provided us not only with inherent assistance in the blood itself, but has also given us the chance to aid it through healthful living, nutrition, and natural juices.

The blood purifying therapy unit consists of:

> 2 bottles stinging nettle juice
> 2 bottles dandelion juice
> 1 bottle celery juice

1 package peppermint tea or
2 packages Floralax Herbal Tea[1]

**1st - 4th day**

Before breakfast:    1 cup water or peppermint tea with
1 tablespoon nettle juice

Before lunch:    1 tablespoon nettle juice in
$1/2$ cup water

Before bedtime:    1 cup Floralax Herbal Tea with
1 tablespoon nettle juice

**5th - 12th day**

Before breakfast:    $1/2$ to 1 cup of water or peppermint
tea with 1 tablespoon nettle juice
and 1 tablespoon dandelion juice

Before lunch:    1 tablespoon nettle juice and
1 tablespoon dandelion juice with
$1/2$ cup of water or peppermint tea

Before bedtime:    1 cup Floralax Herbal Tea with
1 tablespoon dandelion juice and
1 tablespoon nettle juice

**13th - 16th day**

Before breakfast:    $1/2$ cup water or peppermint tea with
1 tablespoon celery juice

Before lunch:    1 tablespoon celery juice and
$1/2$ cup water or peppermint tea

---

[1] In countries where Floralax Herbal Tea is not available, a non-cramping, very
mild laxative tea may be taken as a substitute.

Before bedtime:      1 cup Floralax Herbal Tea with
                            1 tablespoon celery juice

## The Prescribed Juices

Due to its strong diuretic properties, stinging nettle juice is the blood purifier *par excellence*. It stimulates the metabolism, activates and dissolves waste products in the organism, and flushes them out.

Dandelion juice stimulates the intestinal tract, the liver, gall-bladder and pancreas, thereby indirectly reducing congestion and improving the functioning of these areas. Dandelion juice further promotes the activities already initiated by the stinging nettle juice. In an overall analysis, the whole metabolism and elimination processes are streamlined.

Celery juice specifically affects the kidneys and promotes a thorough flushing out of waste products already dislodged through the influence of stinging nettle and dandelion juices. Celery juice further stimulates the glandular functions and thus raises the general energy level.

If aiming for a complete blood purifying therapy with enduring results, two tasks must be achieved:

1. the cleansing process must dislodge all residues and toxins settled in the tissues and bring them again into the bloodstream in order to be dealt with.

2. by increasing the functions of all eliminative organs – the lungs, skin, liver, kidneys, spleen and intestines – the therapy completely flushes out the undesirable wastes.

These tasks will be achieved by taking the prescribed juices for the purification/elimination process, and by continuing with a simple, natural lifestyle. Fig syrup is a pleasant way of keeping the purification process on an easy, sweet note, and an increased vitamin/mineral supply for the body, especially in the springtime, can be provided with acerola juice.

The therapy unit suggested can be beneficially repeated two or three times, and interrupted and/or supplemented by occasional juice fasting days, so that the whole therapy extends to at least three to four weeks.

## Diet

All excessive eating and drinking is to be avoided during the therapy period. Equally, all foods not easily digested, especially those which create a high rate of putrefaction and uric acid in the body (all animal foods), should be eliminated altogether and replaced by fresh vegetables, fruit, grains and soy products. People with a sedentary lifestyle will greatly support the effects of the therapy by scheduling additional moderate exercise (long walks for example) in fresh air. These suggestions should eventually become part of your lifestyle if you wish to maintain optimum health.

# Circulation Therapy for Veins and Low Blood Pressure

This therapy aims particularly at strengthening sluggish veins. Vein walls are thinner than those of the arteries. The latter receive the "pressure" or positive activity of the blood being pumped from the heart, whereas veins need only respond to the "suction" action, drawing the blood back. One could compare the arteries to outer car tires, and the veins to the inner tubing.

The network of veins serves to drain the capillary beds and body tissues of "used" blood and return it to the heart by the rhythmic sucking action of breathing, muscular contraction and valves located in the veins of the legs. Gravity assists the return of venous blood from the head and neck back to the heart, but the blood flow up from the legs runs against the force of gravity. Valves, which are present in both the deep and superficial veins must give an indispensable push, as well as prevent the blood from flowing back to the feet.

We have, generally speaking, two sets of veins: those near the skin surface and those deep beneath it. If the veins near the surface become permanently dilated and swollen, looking like unsightly bluish cords, we call them varicose. This condition is often accompanied by damage to the valves within the veins. Among the contributing factors are infections, poorly oxygenated venous blood and metabolic waste products.

It must not be forgotten that veins, like all other organs in the body, need proper nutrition in order to function properly. To prevent or ease varicose veins the quality of the blood should be kept "thin," that is, easy flowing, free from cholesterol, trans-fatty acids (heat-damaged fats), saturated animal fats and nutrients high in waste which burden metabolism. The diets suggested in the Slimming/Weight Reducing Therapy section *(pages 166–173)* will help achieve this.

Another requisite would be the appropriate natural juices to strengthen the veins and the circulation; in this case, a combination of bean, hawthorn and yarrow juice.

The therapy unit here will be:
> 3 bottles hawthorn juice
> 3 bottles yarrow juice
> 1 bottle bean juice
> 1 package rosemary tea or peppermint tea

## 1st - 14th day

Before breakfast: 1 cup rosemary tea with
1 tablespoon hawthorn juice and
yarrow juice

Before lunch: 1 cup rosemary tea with
1 tablespoon hawthorn juice
and yarrow juice

Midafternoon: 1 cup peppermint tea with
1 tablespoon hawthorn juice
and yarrow juice

At night: 1 cup rosemary tea with
1 tablespoon hawthorn juice
and yarrow juice

Before bedtime:   1 cup rosemary tea with
1 tablespoon hawthorn juice
and yarrow juice

In cases of inflammation of the veins, greater emphasis is placed on the yarrow juice, in order to restore the consistency of the veins themselves. For this, the therapy plan should proceed as follows:

**1st - 4th day**
Before breakfast:   1 cup peppermint tea with
1 tablespoon yarrow juice

Before lunch:   1 tablespoon yarrow juice in
1/2 cup water

Before bedtime:   1 tablespoon yarrow juice in
1/2 cup water

**5th - 8th day**
Before breakfast:   1 cup peppermint tea with
1 tablespoon yarrow juice

Before lunch:   2 tablespoons yarrow juice with
1/2 cup water

Before bedtime:   2 tablespoons yarrow juice with
1/2 cup water

**9th - 16th day**
Before breakfast:   1 cup peppermint tea with
1 tablespoon hawthorn juice

Before lunch:   1 tablespoon hawthorn juice with
1/2 cup water

| | |
|---|---|
| Before bedtime: | 1 tablespoon hawthorn juice with ½ cup water |
| **17th - 20th day** | |
| Before breakfast: | 1 cup peppermint tea with 1 tablespoon bean juice |
| Before lunch: | 1 tablespoon bean juice with ½ cup water |
| Before bedtime: | 1 tablespoon bean juice with ½ cup water |

## The Prescribed Juices

Yarrow juice increases the elasticity of the blood vessels, permitting an easier flow of blood into the smallest capillaries. All this is due to the rich content of the bioflavonoids which also help to prevent sluggishness and effect a normalization in the venous circulatory system.

Bean juice, taken at the end of the therapy, benefits the whole circulatory system through its diuretic effects on the tissue-bound liquid in the body.

For diet recommendations see Heart and Circulation Therapy, page 147.

# Circulation Therapy for High Blood Pressure (Hypertension)

According to Albert N. Brest, MD, and John H. Moyer, MD, "there is probably no bodily function which commands greater attention, or has graver connotations in the minds of the lay public, than does the blood pressure reading."[1] It is also the least understood by the average layman.

To the physician, hypertension denotes only an elevation in blood pressure. The exact incidence of high blood pressure is not known, but no age group is spared entirely. The cause remains disturbingly elusive in most instances. Loss of elasticity of the large arterial walls (as in arteriosclerosis) can be one reason; an excessive constriction or narrowing of the arterioles throughout the body can be another. Kidney disease is the most commonly known cause for hypertension, though the exact mechanism of it does not seem to be quite clear. More recently, the cause of hypertension has been linked to the consumption of artificially hardened or hydrogenated seed oils – trans-fatty acids – as found in margarine and vegetable shortening.[2]

Whatever the causes ascertained by your physician, the naturopathic approach to the restoration of normal blood pressure is the use of fresh-pressed herbal juices. The therapeutic unit consists of:

---

[1] Meredith Corporation, *Family Medical Guide*, p 114.

[2] Highly recommended reading: *Fats that Heal – Fats that Kill* by Udo Erasmus, alive books, Vancouver, B.C. 1993.

2 bottles garlic juice
4 bottles hawthorn juice
2 packages mistletoe tea
45 evening primrose oil capsules

**1st - 16th day**

Before breakfast:

1 cup mistletoe tea with
1 tablespoon hawthorn juice
and garlic juice
1 capsule Evening Primrose Oil

Before lunch:

1 tablespoon each hawthorn juice and
garlic juice in ½ cup water
1 capsule Evening Primrose Oil

Before bedtime:

1 tablespoon hawthorn juice with
½ to 1 cup mistletoe tea
1 capsule Evening Primrose Oil

Hand-in-hand with this therapy *(see Heart and Circulation Therapy, page 145)*, the prescribed dietary changes should be observed and the suggested supplementary juice-fasting adhered to for better results, together with all additional recommendations to stimulate the circulation.

The addition of garlic juice to this therapy is obvious, since garlic juice lowers blood pressure and helps to counteract arteriosclerosis. It also dilates and relaxes the capillary blood vessels.

Mistletoe juice or tea is also a special benefactor to the circulation, bringing about normalization of blood pressure.

This therapy should be repeated several times, interspersed with juice fasting days.

*See: Heart and Circulation Therapy.*

# Female Complaints Therapy

Natural, fresh-pressed cellular juices assist the stressed and weakened body to overcome tendencies against nervous depression, irritability, menstrual problems and PMS. They counteract such complaints in subtle ways. Eventually, they will bring about greater strength and further restoration by purifying, and by supplying healing agents to the overtaxed organism.

The specific herbal juice therapy unit designed for the specific needs of women contains:

> 4 bottles borage juice
> 2 bottles yarrow or silverweed juice
> 2 packages rosemary tea

This therapy also helps in a natural way to relieve physical and psychological tensions often experienced during menstruation and especially at the onset of menopause. Conditional nervous headaches and hot flashes are successfully relieved with this juice combination.

**1st - 8th day**

| | |
|---|---|
| Before breakfast: | 1 cup rosemary tea with 1 tablespoon borage juice |
| Before lunch: | 1 tablespoon borage juice with ½ cup water |
| Before bedtime: | 1 cup rosemary tea with 1 tablespoon borage juice |

## 9th - 16th day

| | |
|---|---|
| Before breakfast: | 1 cup rosemary tea with 1 tablespoon each yarrow juice and borage juice |
| Before lunch: | 1 cup rosemary tea with 1 tablespoon each yarrow and borage juice |
| Before bedtime: | 1 cup rosemary tea with 1 tablespoon each yarrow juice and borage juice |

The purpose of this therapy is to:

1. purify and regulate the bloodstream and the glandular system, as well as stimulate the whole metabolism and alleviate the oppressed disposition.

2. create a well-organized nutritional program with plenty of fruit (rich in vitamins), vegetables (rich in minerals) milk products, preferably natural, unflavored yogurt, and whole wheat grains.

3. develop a balanced way of life, involving physical exercise, mental, spiritual and creative pursuits – giving equal time to work and play, to duty and rest, to others as well as to oneself, in order to achieve inner harmony.

### The Prescribed Juices

Borage juice specifically affects one's frame of mind in a positive, unburdening way. It restores joy and optimism, thereby automatically inviting harmonious functioning of our bodies. This outstanding quality, known even in ancient times, has now been confirmed in recent scientific tests. Julius Caesar appreciated "good-natured" senators, dispensing borage juice before the senate met. Modern psychiatry shows us with increasing frequency how potently our frame of mind and our state of emotion influences the well-being and functioning of our physical bodies. In other words, the psychological and the physical are interrelated and interdependent. Fresh-pressed borage plant and blossoms exert a specific, stimulating effect on the glandular system, which in turn helps you to overcome a "blue" feeling. To put it simply, it cheers you up! In addition, the juice is recommended for blood purification and as a general tonic.

Yarrow and silverweed juices are anti-spasmodic and are most beneficial for relieving cramps and restoring normal circulation. These qualities alone recommend yarrow juice to all women who suffer during their monthly periods.

Silverweed juice, another natural anti-spasmodic, has been popularly known through the ages as "cramp weed." It is included in this therapy for relief of menstrual discomforts.

All organs of the body show us by their interrelatedness that life and illness do not originate in a single organ — we must consider the *totality*. It is understandable that in a holistic lifestyle, nutrition is of the greatest importance, and support of this therapy with natural foods and avoidance of stimulants will greatly increase its long-range results. Sufficient sleep and rest, plus "catering to the psyche's needs," are further important factors to help achieve inner peace.

# Heart and Circulation Therapy

The centre of the blood circulation system is the heart. Every minute it is in close contact with every part of our body through large arteries and veins. By way of this wondrous circulatory system, all other organs and body systems are related to each other, as well as to the heart, and any alteration in the heart's function thus immediately becomes the concern of the whole person. It logically follows then, that the care and healthy maintenance of the heart (our "life pump") and of the whole circulatory system is of the utmost importance for well-being.

In order to better consider specific aspects, the relevant therapy for the heart and the circulatory system has been subdivided into the following three sections: nervous heart and blood circulation, below; therapy for low blood pressure, page 136; and circulation therapy for high blood pressure, page 140.

## Nervous Heart and Blood Circulation Therapy

The therapy unit here will be:

4 bottles hawthorn juice
2 bottles bean juice
1 package camomile tea

**1st - 4th day**
Before breakfast:          1 cup camomile tea with
                           1 tablespoon bean juice

| Before lunch: | 2 tablespoons bean juice in 1 glass water |
| Before bedtime: | 1 tablespoon bean juice 1 glass water |

**5th - 12th day**

| Before breakfast: | 1 cup camomile tea and 2 tablespoons hawthorn juice |
| Before lunch: | 2 tablespoons hawthorn juice in 1 glass water |
| Before bedtime: | 2 tablespoons hawthorn juice in 1 glass water |

**13th - 16th day**

| Before breakfast: | 1 cup camomile tea with 2 tablespoons bean juice |
| Before lunch: | 1 tablespoon garlic juice and 1 tablespoon hawthorn juice in 1 glass water |
| Before bedtime: | 2 tablespoons hawthorn and 1 tablespoon garlic juice in 1 glass water |

No more than 4 cups of liquid should be consumed a day.

## The Prescribed Juices

Bean juice is to be taken during the first four days of the therapy. Due to its favorable mineral content, it effects a thorough elimination of all tissue-bound superfluous fluids and relieves any additional stress placed on the heart and the circulatory system in general. It is essential, however, to simultaneously carry out the diet recommended below.

Garlic juice lowers blood pressure and lipids to counteract arteriosclerosis. Garlic juice is especially effective in its action on the vascular system because is dilates and relaxes the capillaries and blood vessels. It is beneficial in increasing blood circulation and heart action.

Hawthorn juice is replete with phytotherapeutic substances from the fresh blossoms and leaves of the plant. These specifically strengthen the activity of the heart and the circulation. If the heart has been weakened by over-exertion or infectious diseases, or if the heartbeat (pulse) is irregular due to nervousness, this juice is particularly effective. While it is recommended to take the therapy unit repeatedly for lasting improvement, hawthorn juice can also be taken just by itself as a heart tonic.

Additional recommendations for the improvement of the general circulation are alternate hot and cold showers (or underarm and foot baths), light exercise, long walks in fresh air and sunshine, and breathing exercises. Vigorous dry brushing of the whole body skin for a few minutes each morning (the "French bath") will massage the skin, make it soft (by brushing off the dead cells) and bring the blood close to the surface, leaving you tingling and glowing. What a way to start the day!

### Diet Recommendations

The diet during the heart and blood circulation therapy should preferably be meatless and low in salt. Avoid dried legumes, cabbage, and all foods that create flatulence. Eat vegetables raw or steamed, and season them with herbs (parsley, celery, tarragon, basil, onions, chives, dill, lemon). Keep liquid intake low and eliminate all stimulants completely.

If you are overweight, both the heart and the circulatory system are taxed much more, so see to it that a gradual weight-reducing program is followed. A cleansing therapy, such as "Sambu Elderberry Internal Cleansing Program," or the "Lightning Cleanse" page 170, supported by natural herbal laxatives (fig syrup), would be an ideal start, and a few juice fasting days each week will bring you to your goal much sooner. Such juice-fasting days relieve the heart and circulation and increase the effectiveness of plant juices.

## Kidney and Bladder Disorders Therapy

Located on either side of the spine, just below the waistline, the bean-shaped kidneys eliminate from the blood all substances which are no longer of constructive use to the body. The heart and the kidneys are the most important organs of the circulatory/eliminative system. They maintain the "quality" of our blood.

If blood does not flow easily and strongly through the kidneys, due to weakened heart activity, uric acid wastes cannot be eliminated quickly enough. As these toxins accumulate in the tissues of our body, our health becomes impaired.

The therapy for kidney and bladder disorders is designed primarily to flush out superfluous liquids and toxins retained in the tissues by stimulating and strengthening the activity of the kidneys. This relieves the body of the additional stress of coping with unwanted waste material, and at the same time prevents more serious diseases.

The therapy unit consists of:

2 bottles horsetail juice
1 bottle birch juice
1 package uva ursi tea
2 packages rosehip tea

**1st - 4th day**
Before breakfast:

1 cup uva ursi tea with
1 tablespoon birch juice and
1 tablespoon horsetail juice

Before lunch:          1 cup uva ursi tea with
                       1 tablespoon birch juice and
                       1 tablespoon horsetail juice

Before bedtime:        1 cup uva ursi tea with
                       1 tablespoon birch juice and
                       1 tablespoon horsetail juice

During the day, drink rosehip tea whenever thirsty or desired.

**5th - 8th day**          same as above, except **no** birch juice

## The Prescribed Juices

Horsetail juice is most effectively used for insufficient kidney function, for fluid retention in the body and for mild bladder catarrhs.

Birch juice strengthens and increases the function of the kidneys due to its multi-mineral content and other healing properties. It mildly soothes any existing inflammation, is a strong diuretic, and considerably reduces the albumen content in the urine.

The uva ursi tea supports the activities of both horsetail and birch juices, and can be taken alternately with acerola juice to dilute these juices. The latter would also supply the body with additional vitamin C.

This therapy unit can be effectively extended to three to four weeks' duration and, as previously mentioned, should be complemented by interspersed juice fasting days.

## Diet

As in all therapies, raw vegetables and fruit, salads, cereals, whole grain breads, and fresh-pressed unrefined seed oils such as flax, sunflower, safflower, or walnut are to be favored over cooked, heavy meals. Meat and animal proteins in general are to be eliminated at least during the therapy period, and salt intake reduced or completely avoided. Mild exercises and long walks in fresh air will assist both the circulation and the body's attempt to eliminate wastes.

# Liver and Gallbladder Therapy

The liver is the largest gland of our body and is rich in blood. As a matter of fact, it is downright "full-blooded," since it is constantly improving blood quality by purifying it of toxins and waste substances.

A further task is performed by the liver in the manufacture of bile, which is accumulated and stored in the gallbladder for use in the digestive tract. Due to our modern way of living and eating, and the increased pollution in our environment, the liver has become the most overtaxed organ after the heart. Fortunately however, liver cells are capable of considerable regeneration.

The liver and gallbladder therapy aims at assisting these organs in their highly demanding tasks. The therapy unit consists of:

> 3 bottles black radish juice
> 2 bottles dandelion juice
> 1 bottle fig syrup
> 2 packages peppermint tea

**1st - 4th day**

Before breakfast:      1 cup peppermint tea with
1 tablespoon dandelion juice

Before lunch:      1 tablespoon dandelion juice in
1/2 cup water

| | |
|---|---|
| At night: | 1 tablespoon dandelion juice in 1 cup peppermint tea |
| Before bedtime: | 1 teaspoon fig syrup |

**5th - 12th day**

| | |
|---|---|
| Before breakfast: | 1 tablespoon black radish juice in 1 cup peppermint tea |
| Before lunch: | 1 tablespoon black radish juice in $^1/_2$ cup water |
| At night: | 1 tablespoon black radish juice in 1 cup peppermint tea |
| Before bedtime: | 1 teaspoon fig syrup |

| | |
|---|---|
| **13th - 16th day** | repeat schedule for 1st-4th day |
| **17th - 20th day** | repeat schedule for 1st-4th day |

## The Prescribed Juices

Dandelion juice has a restorative tonic effect on the liver. It promotes an efficient assimilation of nutrients and stimulates the peristaltic movements of the bowels.

Black radish juice is an ancient herbal remedy for gallbladder complaints, particularly for stones. It is equally helpful for treating inflamed obstructions of the bile duct. The main healing agents are its etheric oils and its rich supply of organic magnesium.

Fig syrup is a natural plant remedy for lazy bowels. It stimulates the sluggish activity of the intestinal tract, thereby promoting a more efficient elimination. The right dosage is easily ascertained on an individual basis.

153

The therapy unit, as outlined, should be repeated several times for best results, and supplemented with juice fasting days at regular intervals. An appropriate diet, rich in raw, fresh vegetables and fruit, avoiding animal proteins and fats as well as stimulants, will favorably support the treatment. It goes without saying that such a nutrition program will ensure a healthy and properly functioning liver for a long time to come, even after the termination of the therapy.

# Nerve Restorative Therapy

Without the nervous system, man would be doomed to a senseless, motionless, vegetative existence. All that we know, sense, experience and remember about the world around us is conveyed to us by marvellous body cells which specialize in communication. The same cells transmit messages that move muscles, give meaning to this printed page, or regulate hundreds of automatic activities altogether too essential to be entrusted to our wit, such as the heartbeat. These cells with their associated structures constitute the nervous system, a labyrinth so intricate that nothing in the living world – and certainly nothing as primitive as an "electronic brain" – can approach its complexity.

Despite the complaints of many people, nerves never become "tied in knots," nor do they jump, twitch or jangle. Indeed, intact nerves are so deceptively placid that it is quite impossible for an expert with the best of microscopes to tell by a mere inspection whether a nerve is working or not. Their messages are as invisible as a conversation in a telephone wire.

There are different parts of the nervous system, based on a division of labor. The automatic or autonomic nervous system regulates all vital functions of our body, such as the heart, lungs, and peristaltic movement, many of which continue while we sleep. The central nervous system, headed by the brain, includes the spinal cord. The peripheral nervous system connects the central nervous system with the various tissues of the body. Pairs of spinal nerves at different levels of the spinal cord obtain "input" (sensory information) and then "put out" (motor responses) messages transmitted from the brain via the spinal cord. The peripheral nervous system includes the cranial nerves that arise in the lower part of the brain and the autonomic nervous system.

Types of nervousness are as varied as humanity itself. It is quite impossible to make general statements about the care of the nervous system, because here the realms of the psyche and the body overlap. Consequently, treatment must be in accordance with the needs and sensitivities of each individual.

The therapy unit for the strengthening of the nervous system consists of:

> 2 bottles valerian juice
> 4 bottles St. John's Wort juice
> 2 packages balm mint tea

**1st - 8th day**

| | |
|---|---|
| Before breakfast: | 1 cup balm mint tea with 1 tablespoon valerian juice |
| Before lunch: | ½ cup water with 1 tablespoon valerian juice |
| Before bedtime: | 1 cup balm mint tea with 1 tablespoon valerian juice |

**9th - 24th day**

| | |
|---|---|
| Before breakfast: | 1 cup balm mint tea with 1 tablespoon St. John's Wort juice |
| Before lunch: | 1 tablespoon valerian juice in ½ cup water |

Before bedtime:      1 cup balm mint tea with
                     1 tablespoon St. John's Wort juice

## The Prescribed Juices

Valerian juice is taken first to thoroughly calm the nerves. All kinds of nervousness, hyperactivity, nervous exhaustion, nervous cramps of the vagus nerve (stomach, intestines), or nervous headaches (migraine), are favorably and quickly influenced by valerian juice. As well, it promotes sound sleep during which the restoration of the nerve fibres can take place.

St. John's Wort juice is recommended as the ideal natural restorative for the nerves once valerian juice has done its work and soothed them. Today, St. John's Wort cellular juice is considered a specific nerve tonic, particularly capable of strengthening the central nervous system. Some suggest it literally deposits light energy into the nerve cells, thus charging them up.

Interestingly enough, the same healing effect cannot be achieved with dried St. John's Wort herb, proof of the superiority of fresh-pressed cellular juices over herb tea infusions.

## Diet

The diet during this therapy should contain mainly simple, natural, raw ingredients, no meat, be low in salt, and completely devoid of any type of stimulant. A spoonful of natural honey, as a source of sugar and energy for the nerves, is not to be ignored, just as it is advisable to cushion "raw nerves" with a little padding of firm flesh by adding further nourishment in the form of soy bean lecithin: one teaspoon of lecithin or three capsules daily. Also, a daily supplementation of a good B-complex tablet is recommended.

A sensible, balanced lifestyle with plenty of outings in fresh air, sunbathing, sufficient rest and sleep, dry-brushing of the skin from toe to head, will add to better functioning of your vital "communication system."

*Those who do not find some time every day for health must sacrifice a lot of time one day for illness.*

*Father Sebastian Kneipp*

## Regenerative Therapy
### *To raise your all-round energy level*

The living organism does not require the help of an engineer or mechanic to regulate and repair itself. It can do both on its own. This self-regulation could more correctly be called self-regeneration.

Plants regenerate themselves by sprouting new side shoots when a branch is trimmed. Crabs, worms and salamanders grow a whole new part of the body, such as a tail, if it is severed. When we scrape or cut our skin, break a bone, or injure our liver, our body mends the damaged tissue.

Regeneration is an automatic process and while we are still young and growing, it keeps pace with general wear and tear. As we grow older, the tempo of life slows down and eventually the stress shows itself in reduced muscular elasticity and strength, in wrinkled skin, in reduced ability to concentrate, increased nervousness, irritability or apprehension. The causes of these symptoms are varied and usually stretch back over the decades of one's life. The signs often begin to surface in the 40s.

The pure, fresh-pressed natural juice regeneration therapy is designed to slow down this aging process by favorably stimulating metabolism and supporting positive, energy-giving activities of the vital organs: the heart, circulation, liver and the whole digestive tract.

The therapy unit consists of:

> 1 bottle hawthorn juice
> 1 bottle nettle juice
> 1 bottle artichoke juice
> 1 package rosehip tea

**1st - 4th day**  In the morning, at noon and before bedtime, take 1 tablespoon hawthorn juice in 1 cup of water or herb tea.

**5th - 8th day**  In the morning, at noon and before bedtime, take 1 tablespoon stinging nettle juice in 1 cup of water or herb tea.

**9th - 11th day**  In the morning, at noon and before bedtime, take 2 tablespoons artichoke juice in 1 cup of rosehip tea.

## The Prescribed Juices

Hawthorn juice improves blood circulation and strengthens the heart muscle. The basis for rejuvenation is thus established by an unobstructed and well-oxygenated blood stream. A feeling of well-being and greater energy results.

Stinging nettle juice stimulates the metabolism which tends to slow down with age because glands cease to function with former vigor. The diuretic effect of nettle juice supports that of the heart tonic hawthorn juice by eliminating tissue-bound liquids.

Artichoke juice favorably influences blood flow to the heart. The way to the heart is through the liver – the detoxifying organ and central station for all proteins. The liver also has close connections with the skin and the digestive system via the gallbladder and pancreas. Artichoke juice provides strong support for the liver.

This therapy should be repeated several times a year, three weeks at a time. For the support and regeneration of your natural rhythm, juices in the above combinations are definitely recommended.

## Respiratory Tract Therapy — Colds, Coughs, Sore Throat, Bronchial Catarrh

"Breath is life." Not only are animals dependent upon breath for life, but even plant life must have air for continued existence. Life is but a series of breaths. From the first faint breath of the infant to the last gasp of the dying man, it is one long story of continued breathing.

Man is not only dependent upon breath for life itself, but he is largely dependent upon *correct habits of breathing* for continued vitality and freedom from disease. When in a closer harmony with nature, man has no need for instruction in breathing. He simply breathes as a child does. But "civilization" has changed this, and we have contracted poor habits of walking, standing and sitting, which have robbed us of our birthright. The contracted chests, slouching shoulders and respiratory diseases so common today provide ample evidence that only a small percentage of us breathe correctly.

The lungs are situated in the pleural chamber of the thorax, and are separated from each other by the heart, the greater blood vessels and the larger air tubes. Each lung hangs freely and is unattached to anything except at the root, which consists chiefly of the bronchi, arteries and veins connecting the lungs with the trachea and heart. The lungs are spongy and porous, and their tissues are very elastic. They are covered with a delicately constructed but strong tissue known as the pleural sac, one wall of which closely adheres to the lung, and the other to the inner wall of the chest. This sac secretes a fluid which allows the inner surfaces of the walls to glide upon each other in the act of breathing.

The air passages consist of the interior of the nose, pharynx (back of the throat), larynx (vocal apparatus), windpipe or trachea, and the bronchial tree (air passages which extend from the windpipe into the lungs where they break into finer and finer branches like a tree).

An average adult breathes more than 12,000 quarts of air per day. This is not only the body's largest intake of any substance, but the most important to life. The life-giving component of air is oxygen, which constitutes about one-fifth of its volume. Almost all of the rest of air is nitrogen, with minute amounts of several other inert gases. More than half of our body is oxygen (water is eight-ninths oxygen). Ordinary combustion is a rather violent combination of oxygen with various fuels (wood, coal, gasoline) producing flame and heat. A similar, but marvelously controlled, process called respiration goes on incessantly in every one of our trillions of body cells.

We need oxygen to burn food and release energy. Cells in their initial activities use oxygen and produce carbon dioxide. One must be supplied continuously, the other expelled, or else the living machinery comes to a halt in a very short time. Cells do not inhale or exhale (breathe) in the ordinary sense. Physiologists think of respiration as the interchange of gases within the cells. What goes on in our lungs is vital, but it's only a way station to what goes on in our cells.

Air passages within the lungs have muscle fibres, but lungs *per se* have no muscles. They are passive organs, expanded and contracted, much like bellows, by movements of the ribs and diaphragm which force air to flow in and out. The basis for proper breathing – "the complete breath" – is the rhythmic and slow expansion of the diaphragm. The nervous and tense man or woman of the twentieth century mainly breathes with the upper part of the lungs and insufficient oxygenation and incomplete purification of the bloodstream are the result. The blood of someone who breathes poorly is a bluish, dark colour. It lacks the rich redness of fully oxygenated blood. A pale complexion is often an indication of shallow breathing.

The importance of correct breathing cannot be overstated. If the blood is not fully cleansed of carbon dioxide by the regenerative process of the lungs, it returns to the arteries insufficiently purified and is of diminished value to the cells. These impurities will eventually manifest themselves in some form of disease. Lack of sufficient oxygen means imperfect nutrition, imperfect elimination and imperfect health. Good breathers are not apt to catch a cold and they generally have plenty of warm blood which enables them to resist the stress of external temperature changes.

The therapy unit for strengthening the respiratory organism consists of:

> 1 bottle coltsfoot juice
> 1 bottle plantain juice
> 1 bottle horsetail juice
> 1 package thyme tea

**1st - 4th day**
Before breakfast:

> 1 cup thyme tea with
> 1 tablespoon coltsfoot and
> 1 tablespoon plantain juice

Before lunch:

> 1 cup thyme tea with
> 1 tablespoon coltsfoot and
> 1 tablespoon plantain juice

Before bedtime:     1 cup thyme tea with
                    1 tablespoon coltsfoot and
                    1 tablespoon plantain juice

**5th - 8th day**
Before breakfast:   1 cup thyme tea with
                    1 tablespoon horsetail juice

Before lunch:       1 tablespoon horsetail juice in
                    ½ cup water

Before bedtime:     1 cup thyme tea with
                    1 tablespoon plantain and
                    1 tablespoon horsetail juice

## The Prescribed Juices

Coltsfoot juice very effectively soothes the inflamed mucus membranes, expels accumulated phlegm from the breathing tract, and counteracts coughs, irritation and hoarseness.

Plantain juice supports the mucus membranes by its in-depth influence on the whole respiratory system. It is particularly effective in overcoming inflammations.

Horsetail juice, with its high silica content, strengthens the ailing tissues in the lungs.

An extension of the therapy unit to 16 days is highly recommended, combined with several days of juice fasting and a proper diet of fresh fruit, vegetables and salads. Breathing by utilizing the diaphragm must be practiced to ensure a deep, complete breath and full oxygenation and exhalation.

## Slimming/Weight Reducing Therapy

The desire for a svelte, trim figure is not only motivated by aesthetics, but by a desire for good health. Grossly overweight people are much more prone to certain illnesses, such as heart and circulation problems, asthma, liver, gallbladder and kidney ailments.

A well planned, natural weight reducing therapy is rewarding in several aspects. The more you are prepared to actively co-operate and follow the treatment, the more lasting the results will be.

Possible causes for being overweight are varied, but they include:

**Hormonal imbalance:** An inactive thyroid or an imbalance in the liquid control system (lymph and pituitary gland) can so influence the metabolism that fat or water is deposited in the tissues.

**Inheritance** has quite an influence on the fatty tissue distribution, especially in women.

**Overeating,** combined with lack of exercise, is the most common cause.

**Disturbance of the water-level in the body,** mainly due to too much use of salt, can be a factor.

Many of these causes overlap and it becomes necessary to consider the inherent inclinations when planning a weight reducing therapy in order to be able to achieve a realistic, proportionate reduction of fatty deposits.

Only a thorough, yet gentle purification therapy which leads to no unpleasant side effects should be undertaken. Drastic fasting periods, with or without diet pills, are not to be indulged in without medical supervision, since they are dangerous for the hormonal system. Instead, single juice fasting days are recommended. They have a stimulating and regulating effect on the glands and metabolism. With this in mind, three points must be considered in connection with a weight-reducing therapy: proper selection of nutrients, therapeutic support and healthy lifestyle.

All fatty, greasy, rich foods are to be avoided or drastically reduced. This includes margarine, refined oils (sesame, peanut, corn, olive), vegetable shortenings, sausages, meats and fatty cheeses. Butter is the most easily digestible fat for the human metabolism as it bypasses the liver. Therefore, it can be used sparingly. Flax seed oil is recommended *(see below)*. Refined starchy foods (fries, pasta, white flour bread and cakes) should also be eliminated during the therapy, and afterwards used very sparingly. They are too low in fibre and too high in calories.

Proteins, on the other hand, are recommended in the form of low-fat dairy products, cottage cheese, quark, low-fat cheese, unprocessed grains and cereals, as well as legumes which are high in fibre. Seven-grain, whole wheat, or whole rye bread and crisp bread are preferred. No animal proteins other than low-fat dairy proteins are permitted. Buttermilk and natural unsweetened yogurt are highly recommended because of high content of (L+) Lactic acid, a stimulant for increased metabolism. Fruit and vegetables (complex carbohydrates) can be eaten to your heart's content, preferably raw. They are low in calories, give bulk and fibre, thus satisfying hunger pangs and promoting digestion and elimination. When making salads, make your own dressing with lemon or Molkosan (Swiss whey) with small amounts of flax oil (a maximum of two tablespoons daily). Flax oil is rich in the essential fatty acids: linolenic (omega-3) and linoleic (omega-6) which are required for healthy body functions. Most importantly, flax oil helps in fat metabolism, reduces serum cholesterol and blood lipids, which aids in weight reduction.

Predominantly alkaline nourishment, as outlined above, is highly important in a weight reducing therapy to neutralize the acid waste materials that are being loosened and expelled. In this way, auto-toxicity can be avoided.

The total daily intake of calories is to be no more than 1200 calories or 5076 joules. Sufficient fluids of at least one litre (approximately one quart) per day are supplied through fruit and the prescribed pressed juices.

When embarking on a weight loss or cleansing-slimming juice therapy, one can choose a number of different juice combinations for achieving the required results. But whatever combination of juices you choose, you want to maximize their synergistic effect of stimulating all eliminating organs, increasing metabolism and purifying the blood of metabolic waste, while at the same time supplying the body with essential nutrients, vitamins and minerals.

Following are two different juice combinations, both of which have proven most effective and satisfactory in Europe over decades. They are time honored and safe. Preference is mostly a taste decision.

## Herbal Juice Slimming Cleanse #1

The slimming-cleansing therapy unit consists of:

    2 bottles nettle juice
    2 bottles celery juice
    2 bottles watercress juice
    2 packages herbal reducing tea

**1st - 4th day**

Before breakfast:    1 cup herbal reducing tea (no sugar) with 1 tablespoon nettle juice

Before lunch:    1 tablespoon nettle juice in 1 glass water

Evening:    1 tablespoon nettle juice in 1 glass water

**5th - 8th day**    same as above, substituting celery juice for the nettle juice

**9th - 12th day**    same as above, but with watercress juice

**13th - 16th day**    same as above, but with nettle juice

**17th - 20th day**    same as above, but with celery juice

**21st - 24th day**    same as above, but with watercress juice

Follow until a general feeling of well-being is achieved. If possible, every fourth day should be a juice fasting day.

## Herbal Juice Slimming Cleanse #2

The second version of a slimming-cleanse juice therapy has rightly earned the name "Lightning Cleanse." Not only does this internal cleanse program work fast, but right from the start it gives a feeling of lightness, as the tissues are freed of accumulated toxins and metabolic waste.

The extraordinary value of vegetable and herbal juices as a dietary supplement during fasting periods is steadily gaining recognition. The preferable mix, as in the Lightning Cleanse, is herbal and vegetable juices, as they provide a high ratio of balanced vitamins and minerals, combined with a low ratio of proteins and calories, and are both cleansing and restorative. Furthermore, the acid content in vegetable juices is considerably lower than in fruit juices, and there is more potassium than sodium. Potassium promotes the elimination of excess fluids from the body tissues.

During a fast of several days, or even weeks, considerable quantities of fresh vegetable juices are required. Since their home preparation has proven to be cumbersome and time consuming for many, Walther Schoenenberger has responded to the recommendations of modern nutritionists. Fresh-pressed, cellular herbal and vegetable juices in vacuum sealed bottles are available year-round in health food stores. The high alkalinity of these juices prevents the over-acidity of the system so often encountered during fasting sessions. The juices can be diluted in a ratio of one to three, by mixing with mineral water.

The therapy unit, covering a period of twelve days, consists of:

> 1 bottle artichoke juice
> 2 bottles nettle juice
> 2 bottles potato juice
> 3 bottles tomato juice (unsalted)

Contrary to all other juice therapies described in this book – where one specific juice is taken at a particular time of the day for several days followed by another kind of juice taken for the next few days – the Lightning Cleanse is prepared and taken as a mixed juice cocktail.

For at least ten days, mornings and evenings, prepare yourself a delicious drink with:

> 2 tablespoons nettle juice
> 2 tablespoons artichoke juice
> 4 tablespoons potato juice
> 6 tablespoons tomato juice

### The Prescribed Juices

What's so special about this Lightning Cleanse juice cocktail? How does it work? The uniqueness of this cocktail is the specific proportions of juice mixed together for a maximal synergistic effect, where the results of the whole are greater than the parts consumed individually.

Artichoke juice is a bitter which stimulates the liver's essential functions, namely, to eliminate toxins from the blood. It increases the production and flow of bile, thus hastening the metabolic assimilation of fats, and reduces the blood cholesterol level.

Artichoke juice has a liver-purifying and protecting effect, with a similar effect on the kidneys, resulting in an increased feeling of well-being and a new-found zest for life.

Nettle (stinging) juice is a time tested and proven purifier of the blood and the whole system, stimulating the glands and kidneys. Cellular nettle juice mobilizes toxins and metabolic waste and increases overall metabolism, which is also good for the skin.

Potato juice is relatively high in minerals, providing the body with potassium, calcium, magnesium and phosphorus, as well as vitamin C. Any complaints of an acidic digestive tract will quickly disappear.

Tomato juice provides an abundance of vitamins and minerals, particularly vitamins A, B, C and traces of D, as well as bioflavanoids. Tomato juice has an astoundingly rich mixture of minerals including calcium, phosphorus, potassium, manganese and traces of iron, copper and cobalt. This combination, along with oxalic acid and saponin, favorably stimulates the production of digestive juices, particularly in the pancreas. Tomato juice soothes cramps and is a mild laxative.

## Some diet considerations

The Lightning Cleanse is not designed to be a juice fast where you do not eat any solid food at all, so you still want to take a good look at your eating habits. Rigidly counting calories doesn't make you slim or fit, neither is it healthy. What will help you to achieve an ideal body weight that you are comfortable with is the introduction of more wholesome food. Eat raw, unprocessed vegetables and fresh fruits to your heart's delight. Fibre rich, whole grain breads, cereals and pasta are your best choices for a healthy diet. Lactic acid fermented vegetables, such as sauerkraut and red beets, as well as natural, unflavored yogurt are highly beneficial for improving metabolism. Enjoy a little lean meat and fish, natural cheeses, butter and eggs. But cold pressed, unrefined nut and seed oils must be part of a healthy diet. They supply essential fatty acids but do not make fat.

During the Lightning Cleanse you may want to eat very little or you may want to go totally vegetarian, and only toward the end of the therapy introduce lean meat, fish and dairy.

Try to avoid coffee, tea, alcoholic drinks and any stimulants. Instead, drink herbal teas – and plenty of freshly pressed juices which contain a whole array of vitamins, minerals, enzymes and medicinally active and protective ingredients, such as bitters and aromatics. During the Lightning Cleanse your daily intake of liquids, including water and vegetable broth, should be about two litres.

The Lightning Cleanse as a fasting therapy is also indicated for improvement of circulation, chronic constipation, digestive problems, bowel inflammation, skin problems, infectious disease and feverish conditions, as well as for rheumatic, arthritic or gout complaints.

Finally, a word of caution: When juice fasting, it is most important that tomato juice be salt-free, as sodium counteracts the desired effect by increasing water retention within the cells.

An excellent guide to fasting with menus and "fast breaking" instructions is a book by Klaus Kaufmann, *The Joy of Juice Fasting*, published by *alive* books, and available in health food stores.

## Stomach and Intestinal Problems Therapy

Since the digestive organs' willingness to co-operate with other parts of the body entirely depends on what we put into them and how we do it, it is obvious that great discrimination is called for in the selection of our nourishment. In addition, each morsel ought to be properly chewed and blended with saliva before sending it on to the stomach for further processing.

Everything we do for our stomachs and intestines benefits the whole body, because these organs affect the quality of our blood, our skin, moods, mental alertness, as well as the smooth functioning of the heart and circulatory system. No wonder that the physicians' universal question is, "How is your stomach and how do your bowels work?"

The therapy unit, which aims at restoration of these organs to normal function, consists of:

|  |  |
|---|---|
|  | 2 bottles wormwood juice |
|  | 1 bottle yarrow juice |
|  | 1 package peppermint tea |
| **1st - 4th day** |  |
| Before breakfast: | 1 cup peppermint tea with 1 tablespoon wormwood juice |
| Before lunch: | 1 tablespoon wormwood juice in ½ cup water |

| Midafternoon: | 1 tablespoon wormwood juice in ½ cup water or milk |
|---|---|
| Before bedtime: | 1 cup peppermint tea with 1 tablespoon wormwood juice |
| **5th - 8th day** | same as above, but with yarrow juice instead of wormwood juice |
| **9th - 10th day** | repeat schedule for 1st-4th day |

## The Prescribed Juices

Wormwood juice is an old home remedy for intestinal and stomach problems. It is often recommended in cases of too little or too much acidity (heartburn/indigestion). Even headaches and flatulence, caused by faulty digestion, will be relieved by the use of this juice, as its bitter components stimulate the activity of the digestive juices.

Yarrow juice soothes and calms a nervous stomach, intestinal cramps and catarrhs. It restores the normal acidity of the stomach. In cases of ulcer flare-ups, its astringent properties help to seal off the bleeding and soreness of the inner stomach lining.

This therapy should be extended to a duration of three weeks if possible, and combined with an easily digestible diet.

## Diet Considerations

Fatty or heavy or rich foods (salty, smoked meat, highly spiced foods, all legumes) are to be avoided. Several smaller meals are preferable to three large meals a day. Abstinence from alcohol and tobacco should be observed, since these are irritants to the digestive organs.

During the therapy it is recommended to switch to a vegetarian diet. In any case, a simple breakfast consisting of plain yogurt or buttermilk with freshly ground flax mixed in about 10 minutes prior, will assist the fast healing of ulcers, constipation, digestive disorders or any other ailment of the digestive tract.

In severe cases, or when the complaints do not get better, consult a nutrition-oriented physician.

$$\overline{\underline{V}}$$

# Health Cocktails

*The aim of medicine is
to let your patients die
young, as late as possible.*

*Hippocrates (460-377 BC)*

## Natural "Pick-Me-Ups" for Feeling Better

In this segment of *Healing with Herbal Juices* we will look at applications for herbal juices other than the ones for severe illnesses, chronic ailments and degenerative diseases discussed in the previous chapter.

By now you are probably very familiar with the definition of "health" by the World Health Organization: a condition of total well-being of body, mind and spirit *(see page 3)*. We may experience times of extreme vitality, enabling us to do the utmost, such as jumping over fences or pulling out trees. But we also have days when things just aren't "right." No one in his right mind would run off to see a doctor just because of a "run-down feeling," or exasperation because of the "fly in the ointment" which ruins the day. We know that "butterflies in the stomach" before an exam, being "under the weather," or "aching bones" aren't really sicknesses. These stressful feelings are signals our body is sending, trying to tell us that all is not well.

Everyone has his or her own personal physical weaknesses, and, though they may not have developed into the stage where they might be called a "disease," they are not making life very pleasant. Some people experience problems with concentration, others have a hard time falling asleep. Edginess or short temper may plague some people, while others complain about weak stomach, or just plain lack of energy. This state can be described as being neither really sick nor really healthy, just "not feeling well." Cellular herbal juices

179

are ideally suited for taking care of these conditions, no matter what the cause: physical, mental or nervous disorders. To help overcome these weaknesses quickly, a number of different plant or herbal juices may be mixed with fruit juices and a little honey to create a pleasant-tasting "Health Cocktail."

Pure herbal juices without added sugar do not have any calories to speak of, but when added to fruit or vegetable juices, the caloric increase is insignificant. An exception is acerola juice. It adds tartness and flavor, lots of vitamin C but almost no calories. When choosing juices suitable for mixing health cocktails, you may want to select those made from organically grown fruits and vegetables. It is of utmost importance that juices used in health cocktails be free of preservatives.

Some of the following health cocktails are especially suited for children who are plagued by sore throats, coughs and colds, as well as those who complain about stomach-aches or have no appetite. Parents should always keep in mind that plant juices are medicinal and therefore should be given to children only as long as the maladies persist. There is no reason to continue the medication after health has been restored.

Your reason for embarking on a program of plant juice therapy may be to regain health after a serious disease, or to simply improve well-being by strengthening your body's resistance to disease, generally referred to as the "immune system." If you are under a doctor's care, using synthetic chemical drugs or antibiotics, you should under no circumstances decide by yourself to stop using them. Always discuss any decision to discontinue the prescribed medication with your doctor. The final goal of any therapy should be to enable the body to function well *without* drugs or medication. The words of Hippocrates are still as true as ever and are most suited to describe Schoenenberger's plant juices: "Let food be your medicine – and medicine be your food." If you decide to take herbal and plant juices for the rest of your life to treat degenerative diseases, such as arthritis, rheumatism, high blood pressure or even chronic constipation, you should definitely consider a diet change and discuss these matters with a naturopathic or nutrition-oriented physician, naturopath or herbal practitioner.

## The Right Amount

The medicinal doses for herbal juices are comparatively small – 20 ml (about two tablespoons) of herbal juice at a time. Mixing two or three juices together for a total of six tablespoons can be quite effective. For flavor or taste improvements, it is advisable to mix herbal juices with at least an equal amount of fruit juice such as acerola, apple or berry juice, or even vegetable juice such as carrot, sauerkraut or red beet juice. Even lemon juice with honey and water makes a good base for a herbal juice drink. If desired, you may add cold sparkling mineral water and ice cubes.

One important detail should not be overlooked – the following basic recipes merely list the proper amount of cellular herbal juice. Use a large juice glass (eight ounces or 250 ml) and add enough fruit juice or non-chlorinated water and ice cubes to fill the glass. Sit back, sip and enjoy.

For therapeutic purposes, it is best to use natural, unsweetened and unfiltered juices from organically grown fruit and vegetables. Juices from concentrates are not recommended as the concentration process involves high heat, which destroys both enzymes and vitamins. It also subjects minerals to a chemical process which may alter the state of chelation and thus destroy the naturally occurring complex.

You will find excellent fruit and vegetable juices in health food stores, some of which have not been pasteurized in the bottling process. Even lactic-fermented (Eden) juices are very suitable for mixing Schoenenberger juices to make health cocktails.

The synergistic effect of several mixed juices is most beneficial. Health cocktails can be taken up to three times daily before meals and at bedtime.

### Anti-Flatulence Cocktail

That "full-feeling" after meals, accompanied by heartburn, stomach pressure and flatulence, must be treated with a recipe designed to correct metabolic disturbances:

3 tablespoons potato juice (for normalizing stomach activity)

2 tablespoons yarrow juice (an anti-spasmodic)

2 tablespoons black radish juice (to increase metabolism)

Mix with apple juice and two ice cubes. Drink very slowly, sip by sip, three times daily for up to four weeks.

### Beauty Cocktail

This drink is recommended for an improved skin condition where non-infectious blemishes, pimples, acne and other skin disorders need attention. Next to the lungs, the skin is the largest organ of metabolic importance. This "skin care from within" is recommended twice yearly – spring and fall – over a period of three to four weeks each time.

Start the first 12 days or so with:

1 tablespoon artichoke juice

1 tablespoon stinging nettle juice

1 tablespoon dandelion juice

4 tablespoons acerola juice or juice from half a freshly squeezed lemon

1 teaspoon honey

Mix in a large glass with equal amounts of pineapple juice (which contains valuable enzymes) and carrot juice. Both should preferably be raw and fresh-pressed; if unavailable, use unsweetened pineapple juice and lactic-fermented carrot juice. Mix well and serve cool.

After about the 12th day, change to the following formula:

1 tablespoon stinging nettle juice

1 tablespoon watercress juice

1 tablespoon celery juice

1 teaspoon honey

Mix with half a banana, one teaspoon of freshly pressed flax oil (for the omega-3 fatty acids), fill the glass with pineapple juice, add ice cubes, stir well and serve twice daily.

**Note:** A vegetarian raw foods diet, high in fibre, will help to give you smooth, youthful skin. Pork must be avoided if your goal is healthy looking skin.

### Breathe-Easy Cocktail

Nervous or allergic reactions may cause breathing difficulties and interfere with a good night's sleep. This cocktail helps improve breathing in cases of allergies, chronic bronchitis and asthma.

1 tablespoon coltsfoot juice

1 tablespoon yarrow juice

1 tablespoon St. John's Wort juice

Mix in a large glass with 1 tablespoon Sambu Elderberry Syrup and a few spritzers of lemon. Take at bedtime or several times during the day before meals.

### Cough Cocktail for Children

In a mixer combine warm milk with:

1 tablespoon honey

4 tablespoons acerola juice

2 tablespoons coltsfoot juice (it soothes and loosens phlegm)

2 tablespoons fennel juice (helpful for expelling phlegm)

You may want to add some fruit to this cocktail according to the child's taste preferences.

### Diuretic and Prostate Cocktail

For everyone who has problems with uric elimination. This cocktail is also suitable for men over 50 to strengthen the prostate gland.

2 tablespoons pumpkin juice

2 tablespoons horseradish distillate

2 teaspoons lemon juice

1 teaspoon honey

Add sparkling mineral water if desired, mix well, and serve.

### Grippe Cocktail

With the sudden advent of the flu and symptoms of coughs, sniffles and fever, you should to apply the following recipe:

1 tablespoon echinacea juice (immune system strengthener)

1 tablespoon sage juice (perspiration reducing, disinfectant)

1 tablespoon thyme juice (anti-spasmodic, disinfectant)

2 tablespoons red beet juice (strengthens the immune system)

4 tablespoons acerola juice or juice from half a freshly squeezed lemon

2 teaspoons honey

Mix well with apricot-rosehip nectar and drink slowly in small sips.

## "Happy-Go-Lucky" Cocktail

For all those who experience "lows" and feel gloomy or depressed. This cocktail is a restorative for the nervous system and for a cheerful disposition.

2 tablespoons borage juice

1 tablespoon St. John's Wort juice

1 tablespoon Swedish bitters

Using a large glass, add three ice cubes, equal amounts of sparkling mineral water and orange juice to the mixture.

## Heart's Delight Night Cocktail

This cocktail is designed for those experiencing trouble sleeping at night due to palpitations, a rapid or irregular pulse, restlessness and/or feelings of oppression.

2 tablespoons valerian juice

2 tablespoons balm mint juice

2 teaspoons acerola juice

1 teaspoon honey

Mix well and sip.

### Immune Booster Cocktail

One can feel it coming on: lack of enthusiasm, aching all over, feeling sick or just being "under the weather." Treat yourself to a miracle immune booster before meals and at bedtime. Within a day or two you will have the upper hand and feel as good as ever.

4 tablespoons acerola juice

2 tablespoons echinacea juice

2 tablespoons red beet juice

Fill glass with red wine or black currant juice.

### Iron Supplementation Cocktail

This cocktail provides iron for cases of anemia or blood loss. It is especially suitable for relieving cramps in both young girls and women during menstruation, and it is also useful for mental exhaustion and for men who have a "run-down feeling" after physical exertion.

2 tablespoons stinging nettle juice or spinach juice

4 tablespoons red beet juice

2 tablespoons yarrow juice

Mix with grape juice and add ice cubes.

## Long Charlie Anti-Rheumatic Cocktail

For improving the discomforts of gout and rheumatism, especially in the early stages.

2 tablespoons garlic juice or 2 tablespoons birch juice

2 tablespoons horseradish distillate

1 teaspoon juniper extract

2 tablespoons gin

1 teaspoon lemon juice or acerola juice

2 teaspoons honey

Mix in shaker, fill large glass with "bitter-lemon" and add ice cubes.

## Morning Health Cocktail

Start your day with an energizing drink to increase metabolism and to overcome tiredness. It's not the purpose of this drink to give you the adrenaline boost of a cup of coffee. Rather, you will feel fresh, awake and energetic enough to face the day with all its challenges.

2 tablespoons artichoke juice

2 tablespoons stinging nettle juice

2 tablespoons dandelion juice

1 teaspoon honey

4 tablespoons acerola juice or juice from lemon or grape-fruit.

Stir well and pour into large glasses.

### *Relaxing Cocktail*

For a pleasant evening after a day's hard work take this cocktail. It will not only relax your nerves, but will also cheer your mind.

2 tablespoons borage juice

2 tablespoons St. John's Wort juice

2 tablespoons balm mint juice

4 tablespoons white wine

Fill glass with natural apple juice and add a spritzer of lemon.

# $\overline{\underline{\text{VI}}}$

# A Final Word

*Many people died while the herbs
that could have cured them
grow on their graves.*

*Father Sebastian Kneipp*

*The chief cause of failure
and unhappiness is trading
what we want most for
what we want at the moment.*

*Anonymous*

# Perfect Health is Everyone's Right

Doctor Albert Szent-Gyorgi, MD, PhD, the discoverer of vitamin C, states, "Full health is a state in which we feel best, work best and have greatest resistance to disease."

Illness is not normal. Often it is the result of years of poor health habits, consumption of devitalized non-nutritious foods, lack of exercise, stress, destructive emotions, and poisons or toxins of various kinds.

Although genetic disorders and inherited dysfunctions are responsible for a very small percentage of health problems, most diseases are caused by external forces and by the wrong decisions we make in choosing our food, work, relationships, living environment and leisure activities. Humans have been created as a living unity of body, mind and soul. Even thoughts, the product of our mental activity, affect our physical condition just as our physical condition affects our thoughts. Symptoms of sickness tell us we have pushed ourselves beyond a level of healthy functioning, exposing a weakened defense system.

Applying herbal remedies, especially cellular fresh-pressed herbal juices, is the *first* step to restore the body to health from abnormal conditions. "The Lord has brought forth medicinal herbs from the ground and no one sensible will despise them," states Jesus Sirach in the Apocrypha, and the famous German herbalist Father Kneipp adds, "Many people died while the herbs that could have cured them grow on their graves."

Symptoms are the body's signals to which we must pay attention. After the first step toward health, the second and third steps must follow to gain vigorous, robust health which is the normal state of existence for the human race. Vitality, exuberant well-being, and a happy, positive frame of mind should be an everyday experience for everyone.

Achieving perfect health is up to us. We can follow the guidelines set forth by the reform nutritionists of the health food movement, guidelines based on natural, unprocessed and organically grown food, combined with a healthy lifestyle. They include fostering good relationships in our families, in the workplace and in our social life.

Equally important, if not more so, is a healthy attitude toward spiritual growth. Attaining a healthy body, mind, and spirit is a continuous and enjoyable, lifelong process. The longer and more actively you work at it, the healthier you will become.

# VII

## Appendices

## Appendix 1
# Questions Most Often Asked About Cellular Herbal Juices and Therapies:

**Q.** Are herbal juices made strictly from fresh plants? What does "fresh-pressed cellular juice" mean?

**A.** The crowning achievement of Walther Schoenenberger is his invention of bottling fresh-pressed juices as quickly as possible after harvesting, using a very special process. Often the bottled juice reaches the storage room within two hours after the plants have left the field. Harvesting takes place in the morning when the sap flows into the leaves, while pressing and bottling is done in the early afternoon. "Fresh-pressed cellular juice" is the term for a juice which has not been boiled, leaving the cellular structure and chemical composition present in its original form. Heat treatment interferes with enzyme activities and with chelation of the minerals. At the Schoenenberger factory, herbal juices are pressed and then sterilized for a few seconds only using an instantaneous plate heater, increasing the temperature to a maximum 92 degrees Celsius. The juice is poured into warm, sterilized bottles and capped. As the warm juice cools off, a vacuum is created.

**Q.** What is the shelf life of fresh-pressed cellular juices?

**A.** The juices are produced in extremely sanitary conditions and bottled carefully, avoiding any contamination whatsoever. As such, they enjoy a very long shelf life as long as the bottle remains unopened and stored in a dark place. Once the bottle has been opened, fresh-pressed cellular herbal juices must be stored in a refrigerator and should be used up within the specified time of the therapy: usually four to five days. Fresh-pressed cellular juices do not contain any preservatives and therefore stay fresh for about eight days in a cool place, or somewhat longer when refrigerated. However, it is unwise to keep a small balance of juice in the bottle for later use.

**Q.** Are cellular plant juices pressed from organically grown herbs and plants?

**A.** It would be absurd to force-feed medicinal plants for faster growth. Minerals, vitamins, etheric oils, flavonoids, trace elements, tannins and all other medicinal ingredients would be available in much reduced quantities. Standards have been set for medicinal plants to contain a certain amount of active ingredients. Only organically grown herbs and plants are suitable for a natural medicine. Walther Schoenenberger stipulated these guidelines from the outset.

**Q.** Are there any known side effects of therapies using fresh-pressed cellular herbal juices?

**A.** During the last 60 years, millions and millions of bottles have been shipped all over the world. To this day, there have been no side effects reported, and there should be none if used according to instructions.

**Q.** Can herbal juices be overdosed?

**A.** Herbal juices are taken for medicinal purposes in small quantities of one to two tablespoons at a time, usually three times daily before meals. Since their action is much milder than pharmaceutical drugs, and they are packaged in small bottles of 175 ml or less, there is no way a person could overdose. Furthermore, the specific herbs and plants chosen for herbal juice therapies are considered to be non-toxic.

**Q.** As herbal remedies are known to be mild in their action, how quickly can results be expected?

**A.** Fresh-pressed cellular herbal juices have a reputation for giving the best results within the shortest period of all other herbal remedies – better than herbal tablets, capsules or infusions of dried herbal teas. When applied as suggested for therapy over a period of time, improvements can be noticed within days. But it is imperative that treatment is not interrupted and that it is completed in the specified period of time.

**Q.** Can plant juices be taken with other medications?

**A.** Generally yes, but it is best to consult your doctor.

**Q.** Have herbal cellular juices been tested clinically and scientifically for efficacy?

**A.** Clinical testing with double blind tests are usually performed with a group of patients on the drug to be tested and with an equally large group on a placebo. These tests, which can run for several weeks or months, are usually supervised by three physicians and consequently are very expensive to administer. Testing of this nature is therefore done only for drugs which can be patented; no pharmaceutical company would advance the money for a natural product that any individual can produce and sell. However, if any medicinal substances have been well tested for a long period of time, then these ought to be our common medicinal herbs. Anyone who has worked with herbs and used them knows from experience that they work. We refer to this as "empirical" evidence. Yes, herbs do work, and have worked for thousands of years. This we know, but we may not know exactly how or why. Like other manufacturers of herbal medicine, the factory of Walther Schoenenberger employs a staff of scientists, testing the quality of both the raw material and the finished product. Ongoing research into herbal remedies keeps scientists in awe of the wonderful interplay of the healing forces of active ingredients present in plants, such as chlorophyll, vitamins and minerals, glycosides, flavonoids, etheric oils and cell salts, trace elements and many more. Traditional herbology and modern science no longer contradict each other. Phytotherapy – the science of healing with herbal remedies – has gained respect as "complementary medicine."

**Q.** How are herbal juices administered?

**A.** Cellular herbal juices are strong tasting extracts which require dilution with water, milk, soup or herbal teas: approximately one tablespoon of herbal juice to one quarter to one half cup of liquid.

**Q.** Can cellular herbal juices be mixed, for example when two, three or more juices are indicated for a certain ailment?

**A.** If not otherwise directed, several herbal juices can be mixed together. The synergistic effect enhances the medicinal effect of the juice.

**Q.** Where are they sold?

**A.** Cellular fresh-pressed herbal juices bottled by Walther Schoenenberger are available throughout the world. Depending on the individual laws of the country, they are sold in either apothecaries, drugstores, health and nutrition centers or *even* by naturopathic practitioners. The largest percentage of sales is usually through health food stores.

# Appendix 2
# Important Names in the History of Medicine

**Shin-Nong** circa 3700 BC
Chinese Emperor, more physician than ruler, author of the oldest natural healing book in the world based on herbal medicine.

**Hippocrates** 460-377 BC
Reputedly the greatest physician of early times, although very little is known of him. Said to have been born 460 BC on the island of Cos, he died at Larissa, circa 377. Long regarded as "the father of clinical medicine," he is said to have established the scientific basis of therapeutic remedies.

**Theophrastus** (Tyrtamos) 372-287 BC
Born on the island of Lesbos circa 372 BC, died in Athens circa 287. A great Greek philosopher and a disciple of Plato and Aristotle, his work on plants earned him the title "Father of Botany."

**Pliny the Elder** (Gaius Plinius Secundus) 23-79 AD
A Roman naturalist, born at Como in 23 AD, died at Stabiae in 79 AD as a result of the eruption of Vesuvius. He wrote a *Natural History* in 37 volumes, describing the beneficial plants used in his time.

**Dioscorides,** Pedanius circa 30-100 AD
A Greek physician who lived in the first century AD. Born at Anazarba in Cilicia, he was the author of the monumental text *De Materia Medica*, in which the properties of over 500

medicinal plants were described. This work was the leading text on pharmacology for well over a thousand years and served as a basis for all the herbal treatments of the Middle Ages.

### Galen  circa 130-200 AD
A Greek physician, born at Pergamum circa 130 AD, died in Italy circa 200 AD. He was one of the most highly respected physicians of the early days and was regarded as an authority for over a thousand years. Latin translations of some of his work were studied in medical schools until the seventeenth century and beyond. He made an enormous contribution to pharmaceutical knowledge, and some of his "Galenic" recipes are still in use today.

### Charlemagne  742-814 AD
Born at Neustrie circa 742 AD, died at Aix-la-Chapelle in 814 AD. King of the Franks, Emperor of the East, and a legislator, he issued laws called "capitularies." The capitulary *de villis* has been attributed to him, but it is now thought that it was his son, Louis the Pious, who issued this act in 795, stipulating which plants should be grown on royal land, among many other provisions.

### Rhazes  865-923 AD
The most famous Islamic physician of the Middle Ages. Born at Rayy circa 865 AD, died there circa 923 AD. Author of two important medical works, the *Kitab al-Mansuri* and *Al-Hawi*, and numerous other treatises.

### Avicenna  (Abou Ibn Sinâ) 980-1037 AD
A physician and philosopher, called the "Prince of Physicians," and one of the most remarkable men of the Arab world. Author of an encyclopedia, *The Canon of Medicine*. Born at Afshéna in 980 AD, died at Hamadan in 1037 AD.

**Hildegard von Bingen,** Saint 1098-1179
A German Benedictine abbess born at Böckelheim in 1098, died at the convent at Ruppertsberbe near Bingen in 1179. She published two important works on medicinal plants.

**Paracelsus,** Philippus Aureolus Theophrastus Bombastus von Hohenheim 1490-1541
A Swiss physician born near Einsiedeln circa 1490, died 1541, he played an important role at the end of the Middle Ages. Influenced by the Renaissance, he sought new fields in medicine, discovering the importance of precise dosages of chemical and natural substances when used as medicines. Meeting with opposition to his thesis on all sides, he wrote twelve hundred medical, religious and philosophical texts to support his theories.

**Brunfels,** Otto 1488-1534
Botanist, physician and priest, born at Mayence in 1488, died in Berne in 1534. He published the first German book on systematic botany, *Contrafayt Kreuterbuch*.

**Bock,** Hieronymus 1498-1554
German botanist and physician, born at Hedersbach in 1498, died at Horbach in 1554 AD. He was one of the earliest pharmacologists, and in 1539, published the master work, *New Kreuterbuch*.

**Fuchs,** Leonhard 1501-1566
German botanist, author and physician, he translated and adapted the works of Galen and Hippocrates.

**Gerard,** John 1545-1612
British barber-surgeon and herbalist. Published the first English language herb book *Herball or Generall Historie of Plantes* in 1597. Translated from Latin, it became by far the most popular herbal for generations.

**Kneipp,** Johann Sebastian 1821-1897
Father Kneipp, a priest in Wörishofen, gained fame beyond Germany's borders as the founder of the "Kneipp-Kur," incorporating hydrotherapy (the science of healing with water) and phytotherapy (the science of healing with herbs) within the framework of naturopathy. Kneipp was an ardent empirical practitioner, meaning that his teachings were based on his own experiences with herbal remedies. His first book *Meine Wasserkur* became an instant bestseller and was translated into 17 languages. His second book, *Thus Should You Live* and his major work, *My Testament and Codicil* anchored his teachings into the medical-scientific community in Germany, primarily because he eliminated the unscientific exaggerations customary in most medieval herbal treatments. His therapy included plant juices, of which Kneipp said, "I can't emphasize enough how valuable plant juices are for the entire human body."

**Schoenenberger,** Walther 1907-1982
Born in Zurich, Switzerland in 1907, he studied pharmacy in Munich, Germany. During his practicum in Nuremberg the young pharmacist researched the medicinal virtues of freshly pressed juices from herbs and plants. His theory was confirmed by countless experiments and analyses, proving that the fresh plant has superior medicinal value to either the dried herb or the tincture of an alcoholic herbal extract. As diseases bear the name of the discoverer – Crohn's or Alzheimer's, for example – so do therapies bear the name of the originators. Father Kneipp is the originator of the Kneipp Hydro-Therapy, Dr. Heimlich developed the Heimlich Manoeuvre and Walther Schoenenberger is the creator of the now famous Schoenenberger Herbal Juice Therapy. This colossal contribution towards public health earned him the highest recognition of the German government. The prestigious *Bundesverdienstkreuz* (Order of the Federal

Republic) was bestowed on him just a few years before his death in 1982.

*This we know; the Earth does not belong to humanity;*
*people belong to the Earth, this we know.*
*All things are connected.*
*Whatever befalls the Earth, befalls the people of the Earth.*
*We do not weave the web of life, we are merely a part of it.*
*Whatever we do to the web, we do to ourselves.*

*Chief Seattle, 1854*

## APPENDIX 3
# List of Botanical Names and their English, French and German Equivalents

| Botanical Name | English | French | German |
|---|---|---|---|
| *Achillea millefolium* | Yarrow | Millefeuille | Schafgarbe |
| *Allium cepa* | Onion | Oignon | Zwiebel |
| *Allium sativum* | Garlic | Ail | Knoblauch |
| *Allium ursinum* | Ramson | Ail des ours | Bärlauch |
| *Armoracia lapathifolia* | Horseradish | Raifort | Meerrettich |
| *Apium graveolens* | Celery | Céleri | Sellerie |
| *Artemisia absinthium* | Wormwood | Absinthe | Wermut |
| *Avena sativa* | Oats | Avoine | Hafer |
| *Beta conditiva alef* | Red Beets | Betteraves rouges | Rote Beete |
| *Betula pendula (or alba)* | Birch | Boleau | Birke |
| *Borago officinalis* | Borage | Bourrache | Boretsch |
| *Capsicum annuum* | Paprika | Paprika / Poivron | Paprika |
| *Crataegus oxyacantha* | Hawthorn | Aubépine | Weissdorn |
| *Cucurbita pepo* | Pumpkin | Citrouille | Kürbis |
| *Cynara scolymus* | Artichoke | Artichaut | Artichoke |
| *Daucus carota* | Carrot | Carotte commune | Möhre |
| *Equisetum arvense* | Horsetail | Prêle | Schachtelhalm |
| *Ficus carica* | Fig | Figue | Feigen |
| *Foeniculum vulgare* | Fennel | Fenouil | Fenchel |

| | | | |
|---|---|---|---|
| *Fraxinus ornus* | Flowering Ash | Frêne | Esche |
| *Hypericum perforatum* | St. John's Wort | Millepertuis | Johanniskraut |
| *Juniperus communis* | Juniper Extract | Extrait de baies de genièvre | Wachholder Extrakt |
| *Lycopus europaeus* | Lycopus | Lycopus europatus | Wolfstrapp |
| *Matricaria chamomilla* | Camomile | Camomille | Kamille |
| *Melissa officinalis* | Balm / Melissa | Mélisse | Melisse |
| *Nasturtium officinale* | Watercress | Cresson d'eau | Brunnenkresse |
| *Petroselenum crispum* | Parsley | Persil | Petersilie |
| *Phaseolus vulgaris* | String Bean | Haricot | Bohne |
| *Plantago lanceolata* | Plantain/Ribwort | Plantain | Spitzwegerich |
| *Potentilla anserina* | Silverweed | Ansérine | Gänse-Fingerkraut |
| *Raphanus sativus* | Black Radish | Radis noir | Schwarzrettich |
| *Rosa canina* | Rosehips | Hanche de rose | Hagebutten |
| *Rosemarinus officinalis* | Rosemary | Romarin | Rosmarin |
| *Salvia officinalis* | Sage | Sauge | Salbei |
| *Solanum lycopersicum* | Tomato | Tomate | Tomaten |
| *Solanum tuberosum* | Potato | Pomme de terre | Kartoffel |
| *Spinacia oleracea* | Spinach | d'epinard | Spinat |
| *Taraxacum officinale* | Dandelion | Dent de Lion / Pissenlit | Löwenzahn |
| *Thymus serpyllum* | Thyme | Thym | Thymian |
| *Tussilago farfara* | Coltsfoot | Tussilage | Huflattich |
| *Urtica dioica* | Stinging Nettle | Ortie | Brennessel |
| *Valeriana officinalis* | Valerian | Valériane | Baldrian |
| *Viscum album* | Mistletoe | Gui | Mistel |

# APPENDIX 4
# A Glossary of Therapeutic Terms

| | |
|---|---|
| **Adjuvant** | a substance that reinforces the effect of another: e.g. in cases of rheumatism, a tisane of meadowsweet may increase the effectiveness of medical treatment |
| **Allopathy** | conventional medicine |
| **Analgesic** | a substance that relieves pain: parsley, wormwood, camomile |
| **Antidiarrhoeal** | that which combats and arrests diarrhea: garlic |
| **Antidote** | a treatment which counteracts a poison |
| **Antihelminthic** | vermifuge: onion, garlic, wormwood, thyme |
| **Antipyretic** | an agent that counteracts fever: elder |
| **Anti-spasmodic** | a treatment or substance that relieves cramps: yarrow, silverweed |
| **Aperitive** | a substance that stimulates the appetite: wormwood, yarrow, angelica |
| **Aphrodisiac** | a substance that increases sexual appetite and activity: fennel |
| **Astringent** | a substance that causes contraction and firming of a tissue |
| **Bacteriostatic** | a substance which prevents the multiplication of bacteria |
| **Bechic** | a substance which soothes a cough: thyme, coltsfoot |
| **Biocatalyst** | a substance which increases the rate of the body's metabolism (enzymes, hormones, vitamins and trace elements): carrot, lettuce, watercress, parsley, black currant, tomato, spinach |

| | |
|---|---|
| **Carminative** | a substance which relieves flatulence: yarrow, fennel, camomile, valerian |
| **Cholagogue** | a substance which stimulates the release of bile from the gallbladder: artichoke |
| **Choleretic** | a substance that stimulates the production of bile: wormwood, dandelion |
| **Cutaneous** | relating to the skin ("cutaneous infection") |
| **Depurative** | a substance that purifies the blood: birch, sage, stinging nettle, plantain, celery |
| **Diaphoretic** | a substance that causes perspiration: camomile, elder |
| **Diuretic** | a substance that stimulates elimination of water from the body by increasing urine production: horsetail |
| **Drastic** | a violent purgative |
| **Emetic** | a substance that causes vomiting; bitter compounds are emetic in excessive quantities |
| **Emmenagogue** | a substance which facilitates and regularizes menstrual flow: e.g. plants containing essential oils and essences |
| **Emollient** | a substance which reduces inflammation and irritation: flax, borage, plantain, coltsfoot, camomile |
| **Expectorant** | a substance that encourages the expulsion of pulmonary secretions: thyme, coltsfoot |
| **Febrifuge** | a substance which counteracts fever: garlic, borage |
| **Galactogenic** | a substance which increases milk production: fennel |
| **Galenic** | of plant origin |
| **Haemolytic** | that which destroys red blood corpuscles |
| **Haemostatic** | a substance which stops the flow of blood: St. John's Wort |
| **Homeopathy** | a method of medical treatment where minimal doses of medicines are administered |
| **Hypertensive** | that which causes an increase in blood pressure: hawthorn (regulating) |
| **Hypnotic** | a substance or property which has the ability to induce sleep: hawthorn, fennel, valerian |
| **Hypoglycaemant** | a substance which causes a reduction in blood-sugar level: stinging nettle |

| | |
|---|---|
| **Hypotensive** | a substance that reduces blood pressure: mistletoe, onion, hawthorn, fennel, garlic |
| **Metabolism** | the sum of the various processes occurring in the living cells |
| **Mydriatic** | an agent which enlarges the pupil |
| **Necrotic** | a substance that causes tissue death |
| **Oestrogenic** | affecting the female sexual functions: fennel, camomile, rosemary, stinging nettle |
| **Pectoral** | an agency used in the treatment of chest complaints: fennel, coltsfoot |
| **Pharmacopoeiae** | publications containing lists of drugs and instructions for the production of medicines |
| **Phytotherapy** | the treatment of illnesses using plant-based remedies |
| **Polyvalent** | a remedy that cures many different ills: camomile (a "universal cure") |
| **Renal** | pertaining to the kidneys |
| **Resorptive** | that which re-absorbs the blood from bruises: flax |
| **Spasmolytic** | that which relieves and counteracts cramps: wormwood, sage |
| **Stimulant** | that which temporarily stimulates nervous or muscular activity: mistletoe, watercress, parsley, rosemary |
| **Stomachic** | a gastric stimulant: wormwood |
| **Stupefacient** | an agent which produces narcosis or partial unconsciousness |
| **Sympathetico-mimetic** | substances having the same effect as stimulus by the sympathetic nervous system |
| **Synergistic** | simultaneous action of two or more substances in which the combined effect is greater than the sum of each working in isolation |
| **Topic** | that which stimulates or restores vigor to the body or to an individual organ: wormwood, yarrow |
| **Vasoconstrictor** | an agent which constricts the blood vessels |
| **Vesicant** | an agency that promotes the healing of wounds: St. John's Wort, camomile, sage, plantain |

# APPENDIX 5
# Bibliography

Alder, Vera Stanley. 1958-1972. *The secret of the atomic age.* London: Rider.

Blandford, Frank. 1971. *Food preservation & refrigeration.* Wellingborough: Thorsons.

*British herbal pharmacopoeia, Part one.* 1976. West Yorks: Herbal Medicine Association.

Canada Health and Welfare, Health Protection Branch. 1983. *Studies on devil's claw.* Ottawa: Canada Health & Welfare.

Chapman, Esther. 1974. *Biochemistry, the earth's elements & your body.* Wellingborough: Thorsons.

Erasmus, Udo. 1993. *Fats that heal – fats that kill: A complete guide to fats and oils in health and nutrition.* Vancouver: alive books.

Garten, M.O., DC. 1976. *The health secrets of a naturopathic doctor.* New York: Parker.

Gessner and Orzechowski. 1974. *Gift- und Arzneipflanzen von Mitteleuropa.* Heidelberg: Carl Winter Universitätsverlag.

Funke. 1970. *Freunde der Gesundheit.* Magstadt.

Hall, Manly Palmer. 1969. *The mystical and medical philosophy of Paracelsus.* Los Angeles: Philosophical Research Society.

Hutchens, Alma R. 1991. *Indian herbology of North America.* Boston and London: Shambhala

Kaufmann, Klaus. 1990. *The joy of juice fasting.* Vancouver: alive books.

Kaufmann, Klaus. 1990. *Silica - The forgotten nutrient.* Vancouver: alive books.

Kuehl, Ernst D., PhD ND. 1985. *Help your heart with magnesium, Hawthorn and Vitamin E.* Vancouver: alive books.

Lucas, Richard. 1979. *Nature's medicine.* West Nyack NY: Parker.

Lust, John, ND DBM. 1974. *The herb book.* New York: Bantam.

Messegue, Maurice. 1972. *Of men and plants.* London: Weidenfeld & Nicholson.

Mills, Simon Y. MA, MNIMH. 1988. *Dictionary of modern herbalism.* Rochester: Healing Arts.

Murray, Michael ND and Pizzorno, Joseph ND. 1991. *Encyclopedia of natural medicine,* Rocklin, CA: Prima.

Nittler, Alan H., MD. 1972-74. *New breed of doctor – a nutritional breakthrough for total body harmony.* New York: Pyramid Books.

Pahlow, M. 1979. *Heilpflauzen.* Munich: Grafe & Unzer.

Powell, Eric F., PhD, ND. *About dandelions – the golden wonder herb.* Pamphlet.

Schauenburg and Paris. 1977. *Guide to medicinal plants.* New Caanan: Keats.

Schoenenberger, Walther. 1976. *Gesund durch natürliche Säfte.* Düsseldorf: Econverlag.

Tompkins, P. & Bird, C. 1973. *The secret life of plants.* New York: Avon Books.

Tyler, Brady, and Robben. 1981. *Pharmacognosy.* 8th Edition, New York: Lea & Febiger.

Vogel, Alfred, Dr ND. 1991. *The nature doctor.* New Canaan, CT: Keats.

Wade, Carlson, 1976. *The miracle of organic vitamins.* West Nyack NY: Parker.

Walczak, V. Michael MD. *Study on Kervan's natural transmutations.*

Wagner, Hildebert, Prof. Dr. 1982. *Pharm. Biology - Drogen und ihre Inhaltsstoffe.* Stuttgart - New York: Gustav Fischer.

Wegener, Ludwig, Dr. med. 1974. *Lebenskraft durch Pflanzensaft.* Zurich: Volksgesundheit.

Weiss, Fritz, Dr. med. 1988. *Phytotherapy - herbal medicine.* Beaconsfield UK: Beaconsfield Publishers.

# APPENDIX 6
# Useful Addresses

| | |
|---|---|
| Walther Schoenenberger<br>Plant Juice Factory | D-7031 Magstadt / bei<br>Stuttgart Germany |
| Dr. Dünner AG<br>Manufacturers of Vitamins,<br>Food Supplements and<br>Health Food Products | CH-9533<br>Kirchberg Hausen SG<br>Switzerland |
| Flora Manufacturing &<br>Distributing Ltd<br>Importers and Distributors<br>of Biological Medicine | 7400 Fraser Park Drive<br>Burnaby, BC V5J 5B9<br>Canada |
| Salus Haus<br>Manufacturer of<br>Biological Medicine | Bahnhof Str. 24<br>D-8206 Bruckmühl / Mangfall<br>Germany |
| Bio-Nutritional Products<br>Importers and Distributors<br>of Biological Medicine | PO Box 9<br>Harrington Park<br>New Jersey 07640<br>USA |
| Salus (UK) Ltd<br>Importers and Distributors<br>of Biological Medicine | 15 Rivington Court<br>Woolston Grange, Warrington,<br>Cheshire WA1 4RT<br>UK |

# Index

**A**

Acerola, 28, 30, 37-39, 55, 91, 135, 150, 180-182, 184-187

Acidic stomach, 89

Acne, 5, 65, 182

Aging, 9, 27, 103, 159

Allergies, 183

Anemia, 27, 38, 75, 105, 109, 186

Anti-flatulence cocktail, 182

Anti-spasmodic, 27-29, 32, 71, 104, 111, 144, 182, 184, 206

Antibiotic, 73-74, 87

Antiseptic, 65, 77, 111

Appetite, 5, 59, 73-74, 77, 82, 114, 118, 120, 180, 206

Arteries, hardening, of 125

Arteriosclerosis, 27, 70, 72, 79, 93-94, 125-126, 140-141, 147

Arthritis, 21, 27, 48-49, 59, 74, 105, 109, 128, 181

Artichoke, 27-29, 31, 40-41, 89, 91, 160-161, 170-171, 182, 187, 204, 207

Asparagus, 29, 42-43

Asthma, 27-28, 44, 60, 74, 166, 183

**B**

Babies, 5, 57, 105

Back pain, 27

Bad breath, 27, 118-119

Balm mint, 31, 44-45, 156-157, 185, 188, 205

Bean, 28-29, 32, 34, 46-47, 137, 139, 145-146, 157, 205

Beauty cocktail, 182

Beet powder crystals, 96

Beta-carotene, 38, 56, 97

Bile, 31, 41, 50, 63, 83, 99, 152-153, 171, 207

Birch, 27-29, 31-32, 34, 48-49, 128-130, 149-150, 187, 204, 207

Bircher-Benner, 9

Bitter tonic, 62

Black radish, 30-31, 34, 50-51, 64, 119, 152-153, 182, 205

Bladder, 27, 30, 34, 42-43, 48-49, 75-76, 149-150

Blood building, 28, 109

Blood circulation, 70, 74, 77, 128, 145, 147, 160

Blood loss, 186

Blood pressure, 27-28, 30, 70-72, 79, 93-94, 126, 136, 140-141, 145, 147, 181, 207-208

Blood purification, 77, 132, 144

Blood vessels, 28-30, 70-71, 120, 125-126, 139, 141, 147, 162, 208

Blood vessels, elasticity of, 120

Borage, 29, 52-53, 121, 142-144, 185, 188, 204, 207

Breathe-easy cocktail, 183

Breathing, 27, 136, 147, 162-165, 183

Bronchial catarrh, 44, 60, 162

Bronchitis, 57, 60, 70, 76, 93, 183

Bruises, 111, 208

## C

Camomile, 30, 32, 45, 54, 90, 104, 125, 145-146, 205-208

Cancer, 21, 38, 96, 103

Candida albicans, 94

Cardiovascular system, 71

Carrot juice, 5

Catarrhs of the lungs, 60

Celery, 9, 27-29, 31-32, 34, 58-59, 64, 72, 86, 88, 132-134, 147, 169, 183, 204, 207

Cellular plant juices, 5, 23, 25-27, 33, 125, 196

Chest catarrhs, 67

Chest illnesses, 60

Children, 5, 45, 61, 67, 93, 114, 180, 184

Cholera, 70

Cholesterol, 27-28, 41, 125, 127, 137, 168, 171

Circulation, 24, 27-32, 52, 70-74, 77, 79-80, 85, 99, 128, 136-137, 139-141, 144-145, 147-148, 151, 159-160, 166, 173

Circulatory system, 72, 79, 93, 132, 139, 145-148, 174

Cleanse, 41, 89, 114, 127, 148, 169-173

Cleansing, springtime, 77

Cleansing therapies, 116

Cold hands and feet, 105

Colic, 44, 104, 111, 119

Coltsfoot, 27-29, 31, 34, 60-61, 76, 112, 164-165, 183-184, 205-208

Constipation, 28, 41, 68, 93, 173, 176, 181

Convalescence, 28, 105

Cough cocktail, 184

Coughs, 27, 29, 34, 51, 60, 67, 74, 84, 111, 162, 165, 180, 184, 206

Cramps, 29, 32, 54, 67, 84, 87, 107, 111, 114, 120, 144, 157, 172, 175, 186, 206, 208

Cystic catarrh, 29

## D

Dandelion, 28, 30-32, 51, 62-64, 87-88, 119, 121, 132-134, 152-153, 182, 187, 205, 207

Degenerative diseases, 21, 109, 179, 181

Depression, 52, 101, 106, 126, 142

Detoxification, 31, 91

Diabetes, 62

Diarrhea, 29, 41, 57, 81, 93, 101, 104, 206

Digestion, 4, 17, 26-27, 29-30, 58, 69, 73-74, 77, 79, 83, 86, 89, 95-96, 99, 102-103, 105, 109, 113, 115, 152, 159-160, 167, 172-176.

Digestive disorders, 176

Diuretic, 27-29, 31, 34, 46, 48, 52, 57, 59, 72, 74-75, 77, 83-84, 86, 98, 100, 108, 115, 130, 134, 139, 150, 160, 184, 207

Dysentery, 70, 104, 118-119

## E

Ears, buzzing in, 70

Echinacea, 31-32, 65-66, 184, 186

Elimination of excess fluids, 170

Emphysema, 93

Enteritis, 87, 101, 111, 120

Essential fatty acids, 46, 127, 168, 172

Exhaustion, 29, 81-82, 101, 106, 115, 157, 186

**F**

Female complaints, 44, 53, 121, 142

Fennel, 29-30, 67, 184, 205-208

Ferenczi's red beet diet, 96

Fever, 30, 60, 62-63, 70, 74, 87, 95, 128, 184, 206-207

Fig, 28-29, 31, 68, 134, 148, 152-153, 204

Flatulence, 30, 41, 44, 54, 59, 67, 73, 77, 102, 111, 118, 120, 147, 175, 182, 207

Flax oil, 127, 168, 183

**G**

Gallbladder, 30, 50-51, 70, 73, 95, 116, 118, 120, 131, 134, 152-153, 160-161, 166, 207

Gallstones, 50, 54, 62

Garlic, 27-28, 31-32, 69-70, 72, 83, 93, 125-126, 141, 146-147, 187, 204, 206-208

Gastric catarrh, 30

Gastric function, 118

Gastric problems, 77

Gastritis, 87, 101, 111, 120

Gastro-intestinal catarrh, 57, 93

Gland secretions, 109

Glands, 5, 30, 95, 106, 160, 167, 171

Glandular functions, 134

Glandular system, 86, 116, 143-144

Gout, 42, 49, 64, 74, 81, 103, 173, 187

Grippe cocktail, 184

Gum infection, 30

**H**

Hauser, Gayelord, 8-9

Hawthorn, 27-28, 30, 32-34, 70-72, 80, 125-126, 137-139, 141, 145-147, 160, 204, 207-209

Headaches, 30, 41, 44-45, 62, 70, 107, 115, 118-119, 142, 157, 175

Heart tonic, 71, 147, 160

Heart trouble, 30

Heartbeat, 147, 155

Heartburn, 30, 57, 118, 175, 182

Hemorrhage, 120

Hemorrhoids, 109

Hoarseness, 30, 60, 67, 84, 165

Hormonal imbalance, 166

Horseradish, 27, 73-74, 128-130, 184, 187, 204

Horsetail, 27-29, 31, 34, 75, 149-150, 164-165, 204, 207

Hot flashes, 142

Hyper- and hypo-acidity, 118

Hyperactivity, 31, 157

Hypertension, 70, 140

Hypochondria, 52

**I**

Immune system, 30-31, 65-66, 97, 180, 184

Infections, 31, 66, 70, 82, 97, 136

215

Inflammation, 27, 29-32, 34, 50, 54, 63, 65, 74-75, 78, 86, 118, 131, 138, 150, 173, 207

Insomnia, 31, 34, 54, 82, 107, 115

Intestinal worms, 70

Irregular pulse, 185

Irritability, 31, 54, 82, 120, 142, 159

**J**

Jaundice, 104

Juice fasting, 114, 126-127, 131, 135, 141, 148, 150, 154, 165, 167, 169, 173, 209

Juniper, 32, 34, 77-78, 102, 187, 205

**K**

Kidneys, 24, 27-29, 31, 41-43, 46, 48-49, 59, 73, 76-78, 86, 91, 95, 108, 116, 125, 130, 134, 140, 149-150, 166, 171, 208

Kneipp, Father Sebastian, 75, 102, 158, 189, 191, 202

**L**

Lactic acid fermentation, 102

Laxative, 31, 51-52, 62, 68, 89, 98, 114, 133, 172

Linné, Carl von, 15

Linoleic acid, 54, 127, 168

Linolenic acid, 127, 168

Liver disorders, 31, 41

Liver tonic, 40

Lumbago, 31, 54

Lymphatic system, 66, 95

**M**

Melancholy, 44, 52-53

Menstruation, 59, 86, 104, 107, 111, 115, 142, 144, 186, 207

Mental exhaustion, 186

Mental stress, 115

Metabolic disturbances, 182

Metabolic waste, 29, 43, 59, 136, 168, 170-171

Metabolism, 28-32, 42, 46, 63, 73-74, 96, 103, 108, 116, 130, 134, 137, 143, 159-160, 166-168, 171-172, 182, 187, 206, 208

Migraine, 30, 41, 157

Milk, 3, 5, 33, 61, 63, 67, 101, 109, 130, 143, 175, 184, 198, 207

Mistletoe, 27, 70, 79-80, 141, 205, 208

Mood changes, 120

Mouth and throat sores, 104

Mucus, 27, 34, 51, 54, 60, 67-68, 73, 75, 83, 87, 90, 101, 111, 118, 165

**N**

Nerves, 28, 31-32, 54, 67, 81, 99, 106, 111, 115, 120, 155-157, 188

Nervous exhaustion, 81, 106, 115, 157

Nervous irritability, 82

Nervous system, 31, 53, 80, 105, 115, 155-157, 185, 208

Nervousness, 31, 107, 147, 156-157, 159

Neuralgia, 54, 107

Neurasthenia, 111

## O

Oats, 81, 204
Old age symptoms, 41, 109
Omega-3, 168, 183
Omega-6, 168
Onion, 27, 69, 83-84, 204, 206, 208

## P

Palpitations, 185
Pancreas, 73, 114, 134, 160-161, 172
Paprika, 85, 204
Parsley, 27, 30, 86, 147, 205-206, 208
Pauling, Linus, 38
Peripheral nervous system, 155-156
Peristaltic, 31, 73, 95, 153, 155
Perspiration, 100, 111, 184, 207
Phlegm, 28-29, 60, 76, 165, 184
Physical exertion, 186
Pimples, 182
Pinworms, 70, 93
Pituitary, 166
Plantain, 27-32, 34, 61, 75, 87-88, 112, 164-165, 205, 207-208
PMS, 142
Poor digestion, 69
Potato, 29-30, 41, 46, 56, 89-90, 113, 170-172, 182, 205
Pressing of juices, 6
Prostate, 184
Pulmonary catarrh, 59
Pumpkin, 91-92, 184, 204
Purple Coneflower, 65
Putrefaction, 57, 102, 126, 135

## R

Ramson, 27, 70, 93, 204
Red beets, 95-96, 172, 204
Regenerative therapy, 41, 72, 110, 159
Rejuvenation, 160
Relaxing, 28, 30, 54, 188
Renal, 27, 49, 91, 208
Respiratory complaints, 111
Restlessness, 34, 107, 185
Restorative, 29-30, 57, 59, 77, 81, 106, 109, 115-117, 126, 153, 155, 157, 170, 185
Rheumatism, 21, 32, 42, 48-49, 54, 59, 62, 64, 73-74, 77, 81, 103, 105, 107-109, 111, 128, 130, 173, 181, 187, 206
Rosehips, 14, 97-98, 205
Rosemary, 29, 31, 99, 121, 137-138, 142-143, 205, 208

## S

Sage, 8, 30, 32, 100-101, 184, 205, 207-208
Sauerkraut, 29, 31, 102-103, 172, 181
Sedative, 49, 71, 82, 115
Schoenenberger, Walther, 5-7, 22-24, 40, 70, 73, 93, 96, 106, 108, 130, 170, 195-196, 198, 202, 211
Shin-Nong, 8, 199
Silica, 17-18, 46, 52, 60, 63, 75, 82, 87, 91, 165, 209
Silverweed, 29, 32, 104, 119, 142, 144, 205-206
Skin problems, 32, 104, 173
Skin rashes, 54, 81

Skin, youthful, 183
Slimming, 32, 41, 43, 59, 90, 110, 114, 117, 137, 166, 169-170
Sniffles, 184
Sore throats, 32, 180
Spasmodic complaints, 111
Spasms, 29-30, 32, 54, 115
Spinach, 27-28, 57, 105, 109, 114, 186, 205-206
Spleen, 30, 62, 86, 95, 104, 116, 134
Sprains, 111
St. John's Wort, 27-28, 31, 106-107, 115, 156-157, 183, 185, 188, 205, 207-208
Stinging nettle, 7, 32, 108-109, 132, 134, 160, 182-183, 186-187, 205, 207-208
Stomach acidity, 57
Stress relief, 32

**T**

Thyme, 27, 29, 111-112, 164-165, 184, 205-207
Thyroid, 107, 166
Tomato, 29, 41, 113-114, 170-173, 205-206
Tonic, 29-30, 40, 57, 59, 62, 64, 71, 75, 82, 85, 100, 105-106, 109, 111, 116-117, 120, 144, 147, 153, 157, 160
Toxicity, 52, 102, 109
Trans-fatty acids, 137, 140
Treben, Maria, 75
Typhoid fever, 62, 70

**U**

Ulcers, 5, 9, 75, 176
Uric acid, 28, 49, 131, 135, 149

Urinary complaints, 62
Urinary, 62, 75, 91

**V**

Valerian, 30-32, 34, 107, 115, 156-157, 185, 205, 207
Varicose veins, 137
Vein and artery problems, 32
Viral infections, 66
Vitamin A, 56-57, 97-98
Vitamin B, 58, 105, 113
Vitamin C, 14, 28, 30, 37-38, 85, 89-91, 97, 102, 116, 150, 172, 180, 191
Vitamin D, 113
Vitamin E, 209
Vogel, Dr. Alfred, 65

**W**

Watercress, 30, 32, 41, 116-117, 169, 183, 205-206, 208
Weight reducing, 41-43, 59, 90, 110, 114, 117, 137, 166, 168
White blood corpuscles, 75, 132
Worms, 70, 84, 159
Wormwood, 27, 29-30, 32-33, 94, 118-119, 174-175, 204, 206-208
Wound healing, 31-32, 65, 84, 106, 208

**Y**

Yarrow, 27-30, 32, 120, 137-139, 142-144, 174-175, 182-183, 186, 204, 206-208
Yeast infection, 94